AF327491

HOW TO TREAT ARTHRITIS WITH SEX & ALCOHOL

Book Description

This is a light hearted but thorough review of both complementary and conventional treatments for arthritis. It includes new observations on the biologic benefits of sex and alcohol. And it describes new medications that halt the progress of rheumatoid arthritis and explains how each type of treatment fits in the overall management of arthritis.

It introduces the scientific evidence that shows how sex and alcohol reduce the pain, swelling and inflammation of arthritis. Other alternative therapies discussed include some old ones and some new ones that have scientific documentation of effectiveness. These include:

- Capsaicin,
- Glucosamine and Chondroitin Sulfate,
- Ginger
- Omega-3-fatty acids
- Yoga, Tai Chi and others.

And some that aren't supported by scientific evidence, including:

- Bee Stings,
- Homeopathy,
- Copper and Gold,
- Magnets,

- MSM,
- SAMe,
- Radon Mines.

Some that are dangerous, like:

- Chapparal,
- Rattlesnake meat,
- Ayervedic products that contain lead,
- Neck manipulations,
- Medicine mixtures of unknown types.

And others that are amusing or amazing, but misleading:

- Moon Dust
- Earth Dust
- Radon Water, or just plain water with "special" properties.
- Red lights in a box,
- The Battlecreek Combination Vibratory Chair,
- Cider Vinegar and Honey.

This book also explains the differences between the major types of arthritis and the ways each is treated. New medicines are described that actually halt the progression and ravages caused by rheumatoid arthritis. Arthritis is a sexist disease. This implies some meaningful possibilities about its cause and treatment. The book explains what arthritis does to your sexuality and what sex does for arthritis relief. It also explores the biological benefits of alcohol taken in moderation for heart disease and for arthritis.

Editorial Reviews

"Filled with serious advice that tells you what works and what doesn't."

Joyce Onyakaba, MD

"Highly informative and comprehensive book about the multitude of complementary and alternative therapies....The book is about far more than sex and alcohol as treatment options for arthritis patients....His writing style is easy to read....This is a great book for future reference."

**Jo Dewhirst, CEO and Editor,
Lupus Foundation of Northern California.**

"I have read it and appreciate its light-hearted but thorough content."

**Alvin Wells, M.D., Ph.D.
Rheumatologist, Greenfield, Wisconsin.**

How to Treat Arthritis with Sex and Alcohol

And Other
BREAKTHROUGHS
AND
ALTERNATIVES

Carter V. Multz, MD, FACP, FACR

ISBN 0-7414-2347-2

Published by:

INFINITY
PUBLISHING.COM

1094 New DeHaven Street, Suite 100
West Conshohocken, PA 19428-2713
Info@buybooksontheweb.com
www.buybooksontheweb.com
Toll-free (877) BUY BOOK
Local Phone (610) 941-9999
Fax (610) 941-9959

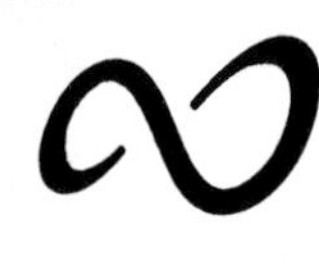

Printed in the United States of America

Printed on Recycled Paper

Published December 2004

Contents

Preface

This book is a revised and updated second edition of the book *Howe to Treat Arthritis with Sex and Alcohol.* It contains much more than a discussion of how sex and alcohol can help in the management of arthritis and the expanded title is intended to better describe the contents of the book. The contents have been updated and the organization of the book was revised to facilitate understanding for those not already familiar with arthritis.

Acknowledgements

To my new editor in chief, my daughter Caryl, I am deeply grateful for kindly, thoughtfully and critically looking over my shoulder. My thanks go also to Beverly Bloss whose encouragement made writing the book possible. I appreciate the kind cooperation of Barbara Erickson for allowing me to quote from her excellent paper about the radon mines. With warm appreciation, I acknowledge the support, encouragement and humor I received from Darlyne Elliott, my patients, my friends and my family. I am pleased and grateful for the author's photograph by Jean Seltsam.

1

INTRODUCTION

During the many years of my practice as a rheumatologist, often patients have come in for their appointments carrying articles and advertisements to share with me. They would pull them from their purses and pockets, and ask me what I thought. Some had merit, but most made preposterous and unsubstantiated claims about unorthodox arthritis remedies. Then my patient and I would talk about it, because I am always interested in what my patients are curious about, and because I, too, am curious about what those hucksters are hawking.

When analyzed, most of these promotional claims were not suitable or appropriate for treating arthritis because they were not based in science, and indeed, most were not even reasonable. That fact frequently had me remarking that it seems we can print anything in this country. And then I joked that someday I would write a book about how to cure arthritis with sex and alcohol. After a good laugh, my patients and I would move on to the issues of the office visit.

After each such conversation, I dropped each brochure and article into a file beside my desk, feeling that one day they would serve a purpose. When the file became stuffed, I started another. On occasion, I would look through them, analyzing them and shaking my head in wonder, and close the file drawer again.

The steady stream of impressively promoted half-truths and hokum really offended me, and one day I thought, *"Why shouldn't I write that book? Maybe the time for this idea has come"*. So I began to research the topic, and what I found is more fascinating and useful than anticipated.

CATs

The emphasis of this book is on therapeutic alternatives, and the focus is on the role of the physiological and psychological effects of sex and alcohol in managing arthritis. These are **complementary and alternative therapies (CATs)**. These therapeutic alternatives do not and cannot replace the essential therapeutic approaches necessary to control arthritic diseases. These diseases are serious and have the potential to be seriously damaging. Don't rely completely on complementary and alternative therapies that are to be used *in addition to* the essentials of therapy, *not instead of* them.

Throughout this book, I will refer to published scientific studies that support the concepts under discussion. The authors of these studies include M.D.s (medical doctors); Ph.D.s (psychologists and other scientists); DOs (osteopathic physicians); DDS or DMD.s (dentists); and some authors who are not doctors but who are contributors to research. I refer to them collectively as "doctors."

Specialists

My comments and suggestions for diagnosis and treatment are necessarily generalized. You must rely on your own doctor for your personal diagnosis and treatment. There are volumes of technical literature covering the subjects reviewed here, so it is impossible for this book to address all of the issues. Rely on your physician for your care and if you can, involve a rheumatologist in your arthritis care.

As a rheumatologist, I am obviously biased. That is, I have had special training and experience, and I am a board certified specialist in rheumatology, the subspecialty of internal medicine that deals with the diagnosis and treatment of arthritis and related diseases. It is the internal medicine side of orthopedic surgery, and orthopedic surgery is the surgical side of rheumatology. In the same way that an automobile driver may not be qualified to drive a truck or a bus, or pilot a boat or an airplane, a physician who is not a surgeon is not adept at surgery, and a non-rheumatologist may not be the most knowledgeable about your arthritis.

Referrals and cost-containment

In this era of cost-containment, some insurers, especially HMOs, may object to specialty referrals. If your HMO or insurer objects, there are valid studies that document the cost-effectiveness of specialty care for arthritis. If you run into this particular brick wall, contact the Arthritis Foundation for supporting literature that will show the insurer that they will save money while providing necessary care more effectively with appropriate rheumatology referrals.

Scientific studies

In quoting studies that support the scientific basis for the physiological and psychological effects of sex or alcohol, we rely on them for the factual information they convey. We do not necessarily endorse any particular activity. The importance of a loving, committed sexual relationship is highlighted in many of the references, and that is emphasized here.

Keep your perspective

In the midst of a heart attack, or immediately after an automobile accident, who among us would ask the paramedics to take us to the nearest herbalist? The role of your complementary or alternative therapies needs to be kept complementary and alternative, and conform to your values. As I quote studies that support the scientific basis for the physiological and psychological effects of sex or alcohol in the following pages, it is for the factual information the studies convey, and it is not meant to endorse drinking alcohol in any form, or having sex. The point I am making is the existing potential benefit of this complementary therapy. If you are a recovering alcoholic, if you are allergic, intolerant, choose not to drink, or have a distaste for alcohol, that's valid, don't drink it. If your chosen lifestyle includes a commitment to celibacy, then sexual relations won't be part of your alternative or complementary therapies, and that's valid too. Also, a secure, loving relationship is an essential part of healthy sex. Casual sex with multiple partners doesn't offer the same benefits. Above all, remember that the products and processes we call alternative and complementary are options. They are opportunities but they cannot replace your primary arthritis treatment. Therefore, take care of yourself, get the best arthritis treatment you can, and keep sex and alcohol in perspective. I guess that's good advice in any event.

Carter V. Multz, M.D., F.A.C.P., F.A.C.R.

November 2004

2

How Do I Know If I Have Arthritis?

Arthritis is a word that means inflamed joint. Many things can cause a joint to become swollen, painful, and inflamed: injury, infection, gout, and a long list of rheumatic diseases most frequently including osteoarthritis and rheumatoid arthritis. Skeletons of dinosaurs show osteoarthritis, and x-ray images of Egyptian mummies as well as the "Iceman" from the Stone Age (the oldest recorded mummified man, one found in a melting glacier in the Alps) show the spurs that mark osteoarthritis. Egyptian examples are reported to date from the reign of Ramses II, the Pharaoh at the time that Moses lived. Osteoarthritis is also remarkably universal. The only mammal that doesn't get osteoarthritis is the porpoise. Whales do get it, so why not the porpoise? We don't know.

Rheumatoid arthritis was first documented in about 1800. It probably existed long before that, but no records have been found that are explicit enough to identify it in earlier publications. In fact, not until the first half of the

20th century was osteoarthritis differentiated from rheumatoid arthritis and gout. Most of our knowledge of these diseases is unfolding rapidly now, nonetheless we know little about what causes them. Autoimmunity clearly plays a role in rheumatoid arthritis, and some evidence suggests that it also has a role in osteoarthritis.

Autoimmunity is the involvement of the immune system in reacting to molecular components of our own bodies. Why this involvement occurs is the basic question behind massive research efforts over the past 50 years. Intrigue with that concept and questions about autoimmunity are what attracted me to the field of rheumatology. Once there, I learned that far from being hopeless, therapy (limited though it was) offered huge benefits to those with arthritis. That changed my course from research to clinical practice. Now our therapeutic armamentarium has grown to highly effective levels.

Each kind of arthritis has a unique personality, which is how we know which type of arthritis we're dealing with. Differentiation is important, useful, and difficult since symptoms can overlap, and two or more kinds of arthritis can co-exist in the same patient. Certain treatments work for one kind of arthritis, others for another, and some treatments work for some, many, or all kinds of arthritis.

Psoriatic arthritis

If the swelling is soft or spongy, not hard and bony, it means there is more inflammation. This can indicate rheumatoid arthritis or one of its variants, such as the arthritis that accompanies psoriasis. Rheumatoid arthritis is described in greater detail in chapter 4. Psoriatic arthritis can involve most joints but it is especially apt to cause severe inflammation of the end joints of the fingers and toes. The swelling can be dense and firm, and it usually has more severe redness and more diffuse soft tissue swelling, and the nails and skin show signs of psoriasis. Spinal and especially sacro-iliac joint involvement are manifestations of psoriatic arthritis that rarely occur in rheumatoid arthritis. Psoriatic arthritis is even more erosive and destructive than rheumatoid arthritis and it resembles rheumatoid arthritis in many ways and many of the medications that are effective for one are also effective for the other. Rheumatoid arthritis also can involve the distal finger joints, but more rarely and the swelling is softer.

Infection or gout

A single, very red, inflamed joint raises concerns about infection or gout. Infected joints are serious and need prompt attention. Gout can involve any joint, but it most characteristically causes intense pain, redness and swelling of the big toe. Then it is called Podagra, a name coined by Hippocrates. Other typical gouty joints include the instep, the ankle and the knee, but it can involve other joints including the finger joints especially in long standing and chronic cases.

If multiple joints are involved, gout can look a lot like rheumatoid arthritis. When there is acute inflammation of a single joint, the main diagnostic possibilities are gout or infection. They look much alike. This can be a tricky differentiation, so if there is any doubt, ask your rheumatologist. Infection of a joint can be very destructive, so appropriate treatment is urgent.

Cysts

Small dense cysts can form near an osteoarthritic finger joint. These bulging synovial cysts are visible and palpable. Attempts to drain them with a large bore needle yields a thick, clear, lightly yellow, jelly like fluid. Under the microscope it contains only a few white blood cells and consists mostly of thick gelatinous non-inflamed joint fluid. The fluid returns immediately, so this painful draining is useless therapeutically but may be helpful for diagnosis.

The most Common Kinds of Arthritis

Osteoarthritis and Rheumatoid Arthritis are outstanding because of the frequency of osteoarthritis and the severity of rheumatoid arthritis. So these will be described separately and in greater detail.

3

Osteoarthritis

Osteoarthritis is nearly universal. Sooner or later we all have it to one degree or another. When I say this in a lecture, there is often someone in his nineties who speaks out to say he doesn't have it. My answer is that he just hasn't lived long enough yet. In reality, he almost certainly has some osteoarthritis but hasn't suffered pain and stiffness because of it, or he is in denial. Osteoarthritis has inflicted every mammal except the porpoise. Maybe someday we can ask the porpoises what their secret is. Even the dinosaurs had it; you can see it in their skeletons. We are more apt to have some osteoarthritis as we get older, but it is not just a function of aging. There is an Egyptian museum near my office and it contains x-rays of mummies that demonstrate osteoarthritis in their skeletons, and they only lived to 35 years or so.

Usually, osteoarthritis first appears late in mid-life. In osteoarthritis, the Heberden's and Bouchard's nodes on the fingers and the often-associated prominence of the base of the thumb at the wrist give a characteristic pattern that is diagnostic by itself. Heberden's nodes are the enlarged, bony, hard swellings of the end joints of the fingers, named after the British physician who identified their significance. Bouchard's nodes, named after a French physician, are similar hard or bony enlargements of the middle joints of the fingers. The prominent bony enlargement of the joint at the base of the thumb next to the wrist is another classic sign of osteoarthritis but it doesn't have a "designer name."

Osteoarthritis can be a "stand alone" or independent process, but it can also be caused by other diseases or conditions. The inflammatory process of rheumatoid arthritis or infection can produce secondary effects that ultimately become osteoarthritis. Trauma is sometimes involved. Sometimes the trauma may be less than obvious, sometimes it is easily attributable to repeated injury or excess use of one or more joints, and often there is no apparent precipitating cause. Football players are prone to getting osteoarthritis of the knees; ballet dancers get it in the big toe. Eventually almost everyone has some signs of it on x-ray even without any symptoms or related history of injury.

In an osteoarthritic joint, there is usually pain, sometimes swelling, and rarely redness. The bones may be enlarged, the angle of the joint may tip to the outside or inside as the cartilage wears away, and an internal remodeling process changes the shape of the joint's bone ends.

Knee joint

When osteoarthritis involves the knee, patients usually complain of pain while walking and often have pain at night. Pain can be a significant problem while climbing stairs, getting in or out of a car, and with many other activities. Swelling is frequently present and can be due to fluid in the joint or simply to thickening and inflamma- tion of the synovial (joint lining) tissue.

Hip joint

Hip joint pain is felt mainly in the groin and may spread down the thigh and to the buttock. Pain on the outside of the hip is from inflammation of the greater trochanteric bursa. The greater trochanter of the hip is the bony prominence to which the strong muscles of the front and outside of the thigh are attached. The bursa, a sack of synovial lining tissue filled with a thin layer of synovial fluid, glides between muscles and bones or ligaments to lubricate and facilitate motion. Patients report the inflammation of this area as hip pain, and indeed it is at the hip, but not of the hip.

Pain across the low back, buttocks or pelvis also is called hip pain by a lot of patients, but it relates to the low back and sacroiliac joints, not the hip joint. Hip pain, like knee pain, can occur at rest, or with weight bearing, or movement, and it can impact weight bearing activities, climbing in or out of a car, or going up or down stairs. Even tying shoes can be a problem. The chairs in my office waiting room and examining rooms are specially designed. They are higher than normal, because patients with hip or knee arthritis have difficulty getting in or out of normal chairs.

Ankles

Ankles or feet hurt with weight bearing and especially with walking on uneven surfaces. The first toe joint at the base of the big toe becomes larger, sticks out, reddens, and hurts. This of course is a bunion, osteoarthritis of the first metatarsal-phalangeal joint (MTP). It is the classic podagra joint of gout, but in osteoarthritis the inflammation is much less severe. But an inflamed bunion can look a lot like gout.

Wrists, elbows, and shoulders

Wrists, elbows, and shoulders also get stiff and sore and lose mobility and function. They can be swollen, but this occurs less often than in the hands, knees, hips, and bunions. Even the temporo-mandibular joint in the jaw can have osteoarthritis with pain on opening the mouth and trouble chewing.

Spine

The vertebrae of the spine are like a stack of blocks with cushions (intervertebral disks) between them. The disks are made of the same stuff as the cartilage in the joints, but the outer fibrous capsule is filled with a jelly like substance, which allows the spine to be flexible. If the disks develop a tear, the jelly tends to push into the weakened area, and if it is near the nerve root, it pinches it. The pinched nerve of sciatica is produced this way. Usually referred to as a herniated disk, this is essentially a breakdown in the cartilage of the spine at that junction between two vertebrae.

A similar process but without pinching a nerve root often develops in multiple levels of the spine, from the low back to the neck. When the disks wear out, the outer capsule tends to collapse and the inner jelly-like center gets drier and thinner. The spaces between the vertebrae are then narrower from top to bottom. The adjacent bone attempts to repair this degeneration by making a different kind of cartilage around the edge of the disk. This is fibrocartilage and it becomes ossified—turned into bone. These ossified repair cartilages tend to stick out from the upper and lower ends of the vertebrae, and they are identified on x-ray as osteophytes, or spurs. This is what you see in the dinosaur skeletons and the x-rays of the mummies.

Along the spine there are ligaments and muscles that connect one vertebra to the next, hundreds of them. They all have pain sensitive nerves in them, and when they are stretched too much, they hurt. The spurs themselves are not painful, and they very rarely cause pressure on anything unless they form too close to the path of a nerve root. The change in the integrity and function of the disks does cause pain by increasing the stretch forces and stimulating the nerve ends in these muscles and ligaments.

Also along the spine there are the normal (diarthrodial) joints, like those in the fingers and the knees. These also can develop the same kind of cartilage degeneration as that seen in the peripheral joints, more typical osteoarthritis, and these too can hurt.

Joint changes

Early in the course of osteoarthritis, changes in the joint are limited to low grade inflammation and very little can be seen on x-ray. Later, radiographic examination provides a valuable tool in confirming a clinical diagnosis of osteoarthritis. The knee is a good example. In the knee there are three main parts: the medial compartment on the inside of the knee, the lateral compartment on the outside, and the patello-femoral compartment between the kneecap and the large bones of the femur and tibia. There are also two special cartilages. The main one is the articular or joint cartilage typical of all diarthrodial joints. This is the cartilage at the end of the bone, like the yellow cartilage on the end of the drumstick of a chicken. The other is the meniscus, a crescent shaped thin gasket that fits around the edges of the joint between the two opposing articular cartilages.

First, one sees slight narrowing of the joint space. This is the space held by the cartilage. There is no actual space in the joint; it is all filled with cartilage and a thin layer of fluid. But the cartilage and fluid are radiolucent, invisible on x-ray, so what you see on the film appears to be space. When the space gets narrower, it indicates that the cartilage is getting thinner. Looking closely, we can also see that the bone under the articular cartilage is denser. Small spurs start to appear. Later, the cartilage space continues to get thinner, the bone beneath the cartilage becomes even denser, and the spurs get larger. Sometimes, especially in the hip, the synovial lining tissue and joint fluid make cysts in the subchondral bone. As the spurs get bigger and the cartilage smaller, the shape of the joint widens and flattens and movement is increasingly restricted.

MRI and CT scans

Magnetic resonance scans (MRI) and Computerized Tomography (CT) scans are rarely needed for diagnosing osteoarthritis, but they can be used to answer special questions if surgery is being considered. For example, the compression of a nerve by a bulging disk can be demonstrated with a scan if it is not obvious on neurologic and orthopedic examination. Sometimes a scan is needed to determine if there is a torn meniscus, gasket, in the knee, but most often a talented orthopedist can determine that clinically, and proceed to arthroscopic confirmation. If required, repairs can be made during the same procedure.

Laboratory tests

Laboratory tests are used to make sure the patient does not have a problem that would make taking medication risky. They are also needed in some cases to review the possibility that some other mechanism may be involved. Osteoarthritis may be a secondary result of other inflammatory types of arthritis. Remember too that psoriatic arthritis, gout, and rheumatoid arthritis can mimic osteoarthritis in some cases, and that two types of arthritis can co-exist in the same patient. Nonetheless, osteoarthritis does not produce laboratory abnormalities, and the *absence* of lab abnormalities, in a way, confirms the diagnosis of this kind of arthritis.

4

Rheumatoid Arthritis

Rheumatoid arthritis rightly deserves its reputation as being the kind of arthritis that cripples. Fortunately today, we have medicines that can halt the progress of this disease and prevent crippling. There are even early signs that with the new treatments, established destructive changes can heal.

Rheumatoid arthritis is not localized to a joint, but is a systemic, generalized disease that involves multiple joints, and other tissues, and organs. If one finds one joint involved, the same joint on the opposite side is usually involved. Multiple joints are always involved, except in some children who may have only one inflamed joint. The joints are visibly and palpably swollen. The pain is observable by a patient's response to palpation, gentle pressure, or movement.

Stiffness

Morning stiffness is a characteristic sign rheumatoid arthritis. While most adults feel a bit stiff after a long automobile drive or for a moment as we crawl out of bed in the morning, patients with all types of arthritis feel increased stiffness under the same conditions. Patients with rheumatoid arthritis feel more severe stiffness and it lasts longer. Even with a hot bath or shower, the stiffness can take hours to wear off.

One measure of how active the disease is at a particular time is the length of time it takes to limber up in the morning. As things improve, the duration of morning stiffness becomes shorter. When arthritis flares the morning stiffness lasts longer. Fatigue is another and somewhat parallel hallmark. When the disease is more active you feel fatigued easier and sooner. Sometimes morning stiffness lets up for only a few hours before fatigue takes over.

Symmetrical inflammation

Symmetrical inflammation of the same joints on both sides of the body is also characteristic of rheumatoid arthritis. In the hands, it typically involves the middle joints of the fingers and the joints at the base of the fingers, but as a rule, it doesn't involve the end joints. Wrists become swollen, painful to move and tender to touch. Picking up a cup of coffee can be difficult. Weakness due to pain and muscle involvement leads to dropping things. Elbows are often attacked. The associated pain, weakness, and awkwardness make it hard to carry things or do normal daily activities. Combing you hair, dressing and eating require elbow mobility that can be lost due to rheumatoid arthritis.

Movement

When a joint is inflamed, it feels better to avoid movement. The tendency is to hold the joint in a slightly flexed position, which, unfortunately, can lead to permanent loss of motion. Maintaining motion is essential, especially in wrists. Since a wrist rests naturally in a slightly flexed position, it tends to get stuck that way, losing the ability to extend. Try holding your wrist flexed, palm down, with your opposite hand. Now, with the wrist in this flexed position, try to pick up a pencil. It will be obvious that your fingers can't work in this position, and that will become a permanent disability if you let the wrist get frozen. Gentle stretching exercises are essential to keep the wrist moveable.

The same is true for fingers, elbows, and shoulders. If you can't move your elbow and/or your shoulder, how can you feed yourself, comb your hair, shave, apply makeup, scratch your nose? Hip, knee, ankle and foot mobility is equally essential. Loss of motion is a major complication, and exercises to avoid it are extremely important. This is a frequent and typical problem in rheumatoid arthritis and other similar types of arthritis like psoriatic arthritis. Loss of motion occurs also in osteoarthritis, but usually it's limited to one or two joints. Maintaining a good range of motion is important in all kinds of arthritis.

Degree of involvement

Many other joints are apt to be involved in rheumatoid arthritis. Knees and hips are the lower extremity equivalent of the elbow and shoulder. Toes, feet, and ankles are like the hands and wrists, except that you need to walk on them, and that can be like walking on sharp stones.

The spine can be involved, including the neck. Of particular concern is the top of the neck, where the joints between the skull and the first two vertebrae pivot and rotate when you turn your head. In some patients these become inflamed, causing the ligaments that hold them in place tend to get weak and slip. If they slip too much, they can lead to serious spinal cord damage and cause paralysis.

If you have neck involvement, wear a brace and drive with eyes in the back of your head, because you won't want to get involved in a rear-end accident. Also, avoid spinal manipulation (chiropractic) to your neck. What I will address again later when I discuss chiropractic adjustments bears repetition here. One of my patients went to a chiropractor for neck pain without consulting me first. As a result of the cervical spinal manipulation, she became immediately and irreversibly paralyzed in all four extremities.

Rheumatoid inflammation in the lower spine occurs but it is rare. I have searched unsuccessfully for many years for a good example of verifiable rheumatoid erosive disease of the spine. If you have low back pain, or even thoracic (upper) back pain, the most likely cause is back strain, disk disease, or the osteoporosis that can be a complication of rheumatoid arthritis and its treatment.

Voice, ears, and jaw

Other joints you may not realize you have, include the crico-pharyngeal joint in the voice box (larynx) where arthritis can make you hoarse, tiny joints in the middle ear that can impair hearing and cause pain, pulley-like joint structures behind the eyeball that can make it difficult to move your eyes, and the temporo-mandibular (TMJ) joints in your jaw. All are susceptible to rheumatoid inflammation. Other things can cause temporo-mandibular joint pain. These include tension with excessive clenching of your teeth, trauma, and dental malocclusion (imperfect meshing of upper and lower teeth). When it is due to rheumatoid arthritis, the treatment is aimed at the arthritis in general, and possibly injection of the temporo-mandibular joint with steroid.

Carpal tunnel syndrome

Another possible sign of rheumatoid arthritis is carpal tunnel syndrome. While usually it's blamed on repetitive wrist motion, in actuality it's due to inflammation of the synovial lining tissue inside the wrist. Injury can cause localized inflammation of this tissue, but so can rheumatoid arthritis. If it happens to be the first sign of rheumatoid arthritis, it can be hard to distinguish between arthritis and injury as the cause. Bilateral involvement can provide a clue, as well as the development of systemic symptoms such as morning stiffness or undue fatigue.

In carpal tunnel syndrome, the swollen synovial tissue fills the space bound by bone of the wrist on the inside, and a tight tendon-like band across the palmar side. This forms the tunnel. Running through the tunnel are tendons, nerves, and blood vessels, all lined by synovial tissue. The nerves are most vulnerable, and as pressure builds from the swollen tissue, pressure on the nerves causes tingling, numbness, and pain in the wrist. Often this extends both distally to the hand, and proximally up the arm. Tapping sharply over middle of the palmar aspect of the wrist where the median nerve runs produces an aggravation of the tingling and pain. Known as Tinel's sign, this is a reasonable test for Carpal Tunnel Syndrome.

Vasculitis

Vasculitis or inflammation of the arteries outside the joint can occur, producing tiny hemorrhages at the fingertips near the nails. In the skin elsewhere it can cause purpura (collections of small purple spots on an arm, or leg, or most anywhere). Around the nerves, vasculitis of the nerve tissue and its lining can produce a very irritating numbness. These are serious signs of systemic inflammation.

Age at onset

Rheumatoid arthritis doesn't respect age. It can begin in infants, children, young people, midlife, or seniors. It is most common in young women, and frequently begins shortly after the birth of a baby. By midlife it is about equally distributed between males and females, and it's more common in men than women if the onset is after age 60. The prevalence of rheumatoid arthritis increases with age, from 0.3% of the population in adults under age 35, to over 10% in persons over 65. It is higher in females than males by a factor of about 2.5 to 1. Pregnancy usually induces a remission, but after the delivery the arthritis exacerbates. The initial appearance of the disease often follows a pregnancy. Menopause is also a time when rheumatoid arthritis is more apt to occur.

What causes arthritis?

Since rheumatoid arthritis occurs so much more frequently in women, hormones certainly play a role, but the exact mechanisms are unclear. Some families have several relatives with the disease, suggesting a genetic pattern. More commonly, families have no history of anyone else who's had rheumatoid arthritis. Identical twins both have rheumatoid arthritis in about 34% of cases, while only about 11% of fraternal twins share the disease. Occasionally, one spouse develops rheumatoid arthritis, and later the other one gets it. Genetics plays some sort of role, but it's not always evident and in many cases any evident genetic factor seems to be missing.

Something else must be involved. Something that doesn't relate to what one does or doesn't do, or eats or fails to eat. Besides the genetic element, which probably determines whether one can develop rheumatoid arthritis, something else in the environment must be involved. I think a virus, or, most likely, multiple different viruses may be to blame.

A virus has the capacity to enter the nucleus of cells and manipulate the functions of genes. There may be several or possibly many viruses that can hook up with the "right" genes to initiate the process that leads to rheumatoid arthritis. And the right gene will vary among patients. Alternatively, possibly cross-reactions between immune mechanisms and foreign proteins from bacteria could cause the response that produces the inflammation that is the heart of this disease. This could even come from immune responses to the shells of already killed bacteria, or to proteins secreted by infectious organisms.

All of these possibilities have been under intense study for most of a century. As technology develops, our ability to see becomes more sophisticated, and our knowledge expands. One of the great things about science is that discoveries are shared and new information in one field can produce new opportunities in others. All the research into cancer, AIDS, transplantation immunity, and even into outer space, opens new doors to understanding arthritis.

Controlling the disease

While we don't know exactly what starts the process, we understand a great deal of what occurs once it gets started. This knowledge is the source of new medicines that are capable of controlling the inflammation in the joints and other tissues. We are in an exciting age of precision. Understanding the immune process has progressed to the level that now we can pin-point specific elements that play pivotal roles in causing the pain, swelling, inflammation, and especially the damage to the joint.

New medicines directed against these kingpins of destruction are halting the damage and dramatically reducing or abolishing symptoms. The new TNF and interleukin 1 blocking drugs are the beginning. New medicines that block the cytokines that cause inflammation and others that suppress inflammation are being tested. These are huge advances. Not only are they thrillingly effective, but because they are so highly specific in their actions, they cause remarkably fewer side effects.

The new medicines are referred to as the biological disease modifying drugs, or Biologial DMARDS or the "Biologicals" for short. The precision with which they work is based on their nature. They are monoclonal antibodies—manufactured antibodies that are directed against one specific protein target. They have only one action, and that is to attach to the protein against which they are targeted. For example, infliximab (Remicade®) is an antibody that attaches to the immune protein TNF alpha, the kingpin of the rheumatoid inflammatory process. When the antibody is attached, TNF can't do its job. This makes it both very effective and very precise. It can't do anything else, so side effects are extremely limited. As with any protein, you can become allergic to it. Anything that blocks a part of the immune process reduces your resistance to infection, so vigilance against infectious diseases and their prompt and aggressive treatment are important.

Development and progression

Today, most patients can be helped in a major way, especially when treatment is started early. To understand how this can be accomplished, we need to look at how the disease develops and progresses.

The initial event in rheumatoid arthritis appears to be activation and/or injury of the lining cells of the blood vessels in the joint. These endothelial-lining cells are much more than a barrier to prevent leakage from the blood stream; they are immunologically active cells that play an active roll in our immune defense system.

Possibly, the causative agent that triggers rheumatoid arthritis is carried to the joint via the blood stream. The endothelial cells swell and gaps appear between them. The tiny arterioles and capillaries become plugged with white blood cells and small clots, and leak plasma into the lining synovial tissue of the joint, and into the joint space. Inflammatory white blood cells squeeze out of the capillaries and invade the tissue. Macrophages, our defender cells, collect there, accumulating around the abnormal blood vessels just beneath the lining cell layer, and deeper in the synovial tissue. In addition to the macrophages, smaller fibroblast-like cells (that make the fiber of scar tissue) collect and multiply. The major immune cells, T-cell and B-cell lymphocytes collect and clone. The endothelial blood vessel lining cells proliferate and new blood vessels form and grow. As these blood vessels grow along with the fibroblasts and inflammatory cells, the lining synovial tissue of the joint grows. It expands over the cartilage and bone and invades them. These inflammatory cells produce enzymes that digest cartilage and bone and this promotes even more inflammation. Inflammatory proteins and enzymes cause the pain, swelling, and destruction that characterize this terrible process.

A systemic disease

Rheumatoid arthritis is a systemic disease in the sense that it involves many joints with bilateral symmetry, and it affects tissues other than the joints. The nervous system even contributes to the inflammation in the joint. Factors are produced in the spinal cord and the sympathetic ganglia and transmitted to the joint via the nerves. Substance P (a neuropeptide) a protein piece that is made in the spinal cord and released by the nerve into the site of inflammation, is one of these. It activates the inflammatory cells, the macrophages and the fibroblasts to produce prostaglandins and metalloproteinases.

These factors are essential to the production of inflammation, so blocking the release of substance P can dramatically inhibit the development of inflammation. Through mechanisms like this, the nervous system probably plays a significant role in determining the severity and distribution of joint inflammation in rheumatoid arthritis. Since the nerves are bilaterally symmetrical, maybe this is why rheumatoid arthritis involves joints in a bilaterally symmetrical pattern.

The lining tissue that surrounds the heart and lungs, abdomen and bowel, muscles and tendons, is similar to the synovial lining tissue that lines the joint. It is the synovial tissue that is the seat of inflammation in rheumatoid arthritis. These lining tissues in other parts of the body can also be sites of inflammation in rheumatoid arthritis. The sclera, the white part of the eye, is related in that the rheumatoid inflammatory process can attack the sclera, along with the iris (the colored part of the eye). This creates serious risk to vision and is considered an urgent medical condition.

Heart, lung, and eye complications

Under the skin, especially on bony prominences like the elbow or knuckles, lumps can form. These are called rheumatoid nodules and they are characteristic of this kind of arthritis. Similar, but harder, lumps form in gout; otherwise, subcutaneous (under the skin) nodules are a specific sign of rheumatoid arthritis. These nodules also can form in the sclera of the eyes and in the lungs. Nodules in the lung may be single or multiple, and on an x-ray they look a lot like cancer or TB, so a biopsy may be needed to tell the difference.

Inflammation can develop in lung tissue that can lead to scar tissue formation, which can impair passage of oxygen into the blood, and exhalation of carbon dioxide out of the blood.

In the heart, rheumatoid nodules can interfere with transmission of signals that control the heartbeat, and lead to abnormal rhythm. Inflammation of the heart lining can cause pericarditis and sometimes fluid builds up in the pericardial sack that surrounds the heart. Fortunately, these heart, lung, and eye complications are rare.

Controllable but incurable

Considering the bilaterally symmetrical joint involvement, the role played by the nerves and the involvement of many structures and organs besides the joints, it is obvious that rheumatoid arthritis is truly a systemic disease. It can also be devastating but with the tools we now have for treating it, we can usually control it or at least reduce the severity. In the recent past, control was much more difficult. Rarely, a patient will fail to respond to the medicines available, but with exciting developments currently evolving, that is becoming progressively more rare. Even though rheumatoid arthritis remains incurable at this time, it is far less likely to lead to severe consequences now. The fantastic growth in our knowledge, fed by advances in technology and cross fertilization by developments in many fields of science, will lead to further breakthroughs in understanding and treating and ultimately curing rheumatoid arthritis and other diseases related to it.

Beyond rheumatoid arthritis, there are many related and relatively similar types of arthritis needing expert diagnosis. These descriptions of osteoarthritis and rheumatoid arthritis, the most common types of arthritis, are intended to provide insight and should lead, if they fit, to a visit to your rheumatologist.

From my perspective

Arthritis is serious, it wears many faces, it's sneaky, destructive, and when you notice joint pain (especially if there is swelling with it), the sooner you seek help, the better your chances are of keeping it in check and minimizing the damage. Find a rheumatologist, or ask your primary physician to refer you to one, and find out what you need to know and do.

5

Arthritis is a Sexist Disease

"Eunuchs do not take the gout," said Hippocrates, and it's still true.

It used to be that gout was 20 times more frequent in men than women, but with lifestyle changes, the effects of some drugs, and increasing longevity, it's now estimated to occur only seven times more often in men. Women are more apt to have rheumatoid arthritis, but the combination of gout and rheumatoid arthritis in women is rare.

Until the mid 1960s, concurrent gout and rheumatoid arthritis were thought never to occur. The combination does occur, but it's rare. During my tour of duty at Walter Reed Army Medical Center, I knew a patient who had both diseases, which can look a lot alike, and misdiagnosis would be easy.

Gout can look like rheumatoid arthritis, making nodules made of tophaceous crystals of uric acid that look like rheumatoid nodules. To find a patient who had biopsy-proved rheumatoid arthritis with classic rheumatoid nodules, and whose joints contained the sharp needlelike characteristic crystals of sodium urate at the same time, had never been reported before the mid-1960s. Shortly after my encounter with this patient, another patient was reported from another center.

Ankylosing Spondylitis

Ankylosing Spondylitis is a rheumatoid-like arthritis that tends to involve principally the spine, and then the larger joints, and occasionally other peripheral joints. It occurs three times more often in men than in women. Related diseases are Reiter's syndrome, and psoriatic arthritis, which occur equally in men and women.

Rheumatoid arthritis and osteoarthritis

By contrast, women are predisposed to rheumatoid arthritis and osteoarthritis. When rheumatoid arthritis begins early in adult life, it is typically a woman's disease. In the middle years, between about 40 and 60, it is more or less evenly balanced between men and women. If the onset of rheumatoid arthritis occurs after 60, it is more typically in a male. Are waning male hormones and the predominance of female hormones the explanation? They may be, at least in part.

Estrogen and testosterone

Osteoarthritis occurs four times more often in women than in men. Polymyalgia rheumatica is twice as common in women. Systemic lupus is 6-10 times as common in women, and fibromyalgia 8-9 times as common in women. Osteoporosis (which is not arthritis but often a complication of arthritis), is also 3-5 times more common in women than men. A.T. Massey reviewed the relation-ship of sex hormones to rheumatoid arthritis. He explained that the sex hormones estrogen and testosterone, and their derivatives, are steroids produced predominantly by the ovaries, testes, and adrenal glands. Corticosteroids derivatives are also adrenal steroids. While corticosteroids levels remain stable throughout life, the production and serum levels of the sex steroids vary greatly from fetal development to childhood, adolescence, young adulthood, middle age, and senescence.

Arthritis is a Sexist Disease
FEMALE TO MALE RATIOS

- OSTEOARTHRITIS   1.5-4:1
- OSTEOPOROSIS   3-5:1
- POLYMYALGIA RHEUMATICA   2:1
- RHEUMATOID ARTHRITIS   2-4:1
- SYSTEMIC LUPUS   6-10:1
- FIBROMYALGIA   9:1

DHEA (dehydroepiandrosterone) is a popular alternative therapy for arthritis. It is a weak male hormone mainly secreted by the adrenal glands in both men and women. Its measurement indicates the level of adrenal androgen production, and it decreases with aging.

Testosterone blood levels vary considerably with age and sex. The difference between males and females begins in adolescence, it reaches its maximum in young adulthood, and then declines with age. About half of the testosterone in adult women is produced by a combination of the adrenal glands (25%) and ovaries (25%). The remainder is derived from precursors like DHEA, which are mainly produced in the adrenal glands. In men, essentially all of the testosterone is produced in the testes. Testosterone is then converted to its most potent form, dihydrotestosterone (DHT) in the cells of the target tissues in both men and women.

Estradiol (E2) is the most potent form of estrogen. In women the ovary produces about 90 percent of the estradiol. Blood levels of estradiol decrease during menopause and with aging. In males, the testes secrete a small amount of estradiol, while more is converted from testosterone in the tissues. Other hormones, including progestogens and androgens modulate the effects of estrogen. It is the relative balance of these compounds that results in the estrogenicity or androgenicity of the overall effect. Beyond this, sex hormone receptors inside the cells can vary and may cause different degrees of resistance to androgens.

Studies of sex steroid levels and rheumatoid arthritis found no significant difference between rheumatoid arthritis and control subjects. A study in males showed similar levels in 14 men with rheumatoid arthritis and 8 with osteoarthritis. Variable findings were reported in studies of androgen levels, DHEA, and testosterone in premenopausal women. Overall there appears to be no significant difference in androgen levels between the premenopausal women with rheumatoid arthritis, and in controls. Similarly, variable and non-supporting findings have been reported in multiple studies of androgens in postmenopausal women with and without rheumatoid arthritis.

Serum androgen in males also produced insignificant, conflicting, and contradicting differences between those with rheumatoid arthritis and those with osteoarthritis.

TESTOSTERONE AND ESTROGEN

Male testosterone decreases with age.

- Risk of rheumatoid arthritis increases with age in men.

Estrogen is highest in young women.

- Risk of rheumatoid arthritis is greatest in young women.

Rheumatoid arthritis remits during pregnancy and flares after delivery.

- Estrogen levels are highest during pregnancy.

Lupus and birth control pills

Pregnancy is characterized by increased estradiol, a steroid produced by the ovary and possessing estrogenic properties and it sometimes can induce increased disease activity in systemic lupus erythematosus patients. In contrast, significant improvement is usually seen in rheumatoid arthritis during pregnancy. Birth control pills more or less mimic the hormones of pregnancy.

One of my patients insisted that her rheumatoid arthritis was suppressed by an early version of a birth control pill. The earlier versions contained larger amounts of estrogens. At first I was very dubious. She demonstrated the relationship by first omitting the birth control pill and presenting increased joint swelling and tenderness, and then reversing the process on resuming the pill. She repeated this little experiment twice to convince me. It was clearly the case, and impressively so. Postpartum flares of rheumatoid arthritis or lupus are also common. Serum estradiol levels show no essential difference between rheumatoid arthritis and control subjects.

In one uncontrolled clinical trial, seven male patients with rheumatoid arthritis were given testosterone by mouth three times a day for six months. Their arthritis was improved by about 60 percent at the end of this study.

Atherosclerotic heart disease in women

Arthritis is sexist in another way. Patients with arthritis, especially women, have an increased risk of atherosclerotic heart disease. Rheumatoid arthritis and lupus are associated with increased hardening of the arteries. Estrogen is thrombogenic. That is to say that it promotes clotting. The cholesterol plaque in the arteries is promoted by the same inflammatory mechanisms in the artery wall as those that operate to cause damage in the joints. Inflammation of the cholesterol deposits makes them grow into calcified, irregular thickened plaques. The resultant narrowing of the arteries is then the site for an increased risk of clotting. So, women with arthritis have increased risk of heart attacks and stroke due to their estrogen levels, their femininity.

Statins, the drugs that are used to reduce cholesterol levels have recently been found to have anti-rheumatoid effects as well. An investigation was started to test whether statins would reduce the occurrence of arteriosclerosis, hardening of the arteries, in newly transplanted hearts. But what they found was that the patients on the statins had far fewer tissue rejections. Further study shows that they are immunosuppressive, and therefore anti-inflammatory.

My perspective

We are increasingly aware of the significance of gender and susceptibility to arthritis and related diseases, as well as the increased risks of cardiovascular disease associated with these arthritic diseases, especially for women. These are some of the ways sex relates to arthritis.

6

Adjusting to Living With Arthritis

One woman told me that she responded with disbelief when she was first told she had rheumatoid arthritis. She had been involved in a rear-end automobile collision and complained of neck pain that prevented her from moving her neck. She consulted a chiropractor who said that her neck moved more like she had rheumatoid arthritis than a neck injury and advised her to see a rheumatologist. At first she wouldn't accept the possibility of such a diagnosis, but over the course of the next year she experienced a slow, gradual onset of arthritis. When her feet began to swell, she made an appointment with me and I confirmed the diagnosis. She became depressed, she said, but was "in too much agony to be angry."

Another of my patients, a brick-layer and contractor, was used to heavy work and loved it. He began having pain in his wrists, which initially doctors attributed to a work related injury. Several different physicians were consulted over many months, but relief eluded him. When he saw me and I diagnosed rheumatoid arthritis, he felt relieved.

He was grateful to have found someone who could tell him why he was having trouble, who knew about the disease, and how to manage it. Several years passed, and despite the best disease-modifying, remission-inducing medications available at that time, his arthritis gradually worsened. Then, when he could no longer work, he became depressed. Now, several years later, he says he remains depressed and is treated for it because, "I am no longer able to do the things I want."

A truck driver said depression was his emotional response to learning he has rheumatoid arthritis. Despite improvement on treatment with the TNF blocker infliximab (Remicade℞), he remains depressed. Why? Because of function loss and pain. He described a recent experience when he had trouble removing the top from his coffee cup. Despite his embarrassment as other truck drivers ridiculed him, he kept working at it until he succeeded because, "I really wanted that cup of coffee."

He attributes his depression to the arthritis pain. "The pain is constant. Pain is depressing. It wears on your sense of humor." However, he also had a background of depression fed by an abusive mother who was the source of two skull fractures. His depression also relates to the loss first of his brother to murder, and later of a sister who died after years as a paraplegic from a gunshot wound to the spine. He requires antidepressant medication, but keeps up a façade of good humor that probably helps him stay positive. Depression aggravates arthritis, and arthritis aggravates depression, but with relief due to the Remicade℞, and his own efforts to maintain a sense of humor, he is doing better.

Weathering an unwanted diagnosis

Most patients today tend to take an arthritis diagnosis in stride. People now are more knowledgeable about arthritis, and it is readily controlled with the therapies available, so the previous response of devastation because of the diagnosis is seen less often. Nonetheless, chronic pain and swelling, fear of deformity and functional impairment, and anxiety about needing to take medications long term can be distressing.

Often depression is an early and acute response to learning one has a chronic, incurable, painful, and disabling disease. This depression can easily become chronic and persistent. When depression persists, it exacerbates and magnifies the disabling and discomforting aspects of arthritis. Antidepressants are helpful, but adopting a positive attitude works better.

Denial

When confronted by an unwanted diagnosis, many patients retreat into denial and either play down or ignore the disease, or seek second opinions. Generations ago denial in the face of hardship was considered strength, but today denial of arthritis can be self-destructive. Seeking a second opinion is fine, if the second opinion comes from a knowledgeable physician, preferably a rheumatologist. To know that rheumatologists have dedicated their lives to helping people with arthritis gives patients comfort, as it should. As for the rheumatologists, no one could survive a lifetime of work in a field of medical specialty without experiencing success often and regularly. I know I couldn't spend my life doing this work if I wasn't used to winning.

If denial levels are extreme, treatment is delayed, and this can do real harm by allowing the arthritic process to advance unchecked. One form that denial takes is the refusal to take medications for arthritis. Pain and swelling are symptoms that demand attention. Alternative and fraudulent solutions may replace more effective treatment when people try special promotions that promise relief by alternative products or methods. Sometimes people travel long distances to access alternative therapies that may not be legitimate. Remember always that alternative therapies are to be used "also, not instead of."

For example, at least two clinics in Mexico were popular for many years because they offered dramatic relief while vowing that they used only safe, pure, natural products that didn't involve corticosteroid drugs. Patients reported waiting in long lines, and each was given the same set of pills, which they then took and felt dramatically better. However, sometimes side effects developed that required hospitalization.

The pills were sent for analysis, which revealed that one of them was prednisone, a corticosteroid. Another of the pills usually was a tranquilizer, most often diazepam (Valium®). Often a third pill, described as tan in color, contained what appeared to be simply dirt from local fields. Beyond the fraud and risk of receiving potent medicines without proper precautions and follow-up, patients failed to receive the therapy that could control their arthritis. What happened instead of relief was increased disease progression, joint destruction by inflammation, and crippling. This is even more critical now that we have access to TNF-blocking drugs that actually halt the progression of joint destruction. Denial is not a friend or a virtue.

Anger and depression

After denial comes anger and depression. "Why should I get arthritis? What did I do to deserve this?" Depression can be serious. Patients may feel hopeless, like life has lost its shine and there's no future. One of my patients became very depressed by her divorce and the arthritis that followed it. She attributed the onset of arthritis to the emotional stress of the divorce, and she wasn't wrong; stressful events can trigger the onset of rheumatoid arthritis or systemic lupus. My patient had a vibrating recliner that she loved because it gave her some relief from her arthritis. One day, she settled into that favorite chair and shot and killed herself. In her will she expressed appreciation for my help in her treatment, and she willed that chair to me.

Eventually, most patients with arthritis experience emotional growth to a level rarely reached by the rest of us as they come to terms with the disease and decide they won't let arthritis ruin their lives. They choose to decide how they will live their lives, and not let disease make the decision for them. They become more understanding, thoughtful, tolerant of others, and they are wonderful to know and work with.

Attitude matters

She was one of my favorite people. I'll call her Margaret. She was a receptionist-PBX telephone operator at the Robert Breck Brigham hospital in Boston, now part of the Brigham and Women's Hospital. The Robert Brigham, a hospital dedicated to the study and treatment of arthritis, was where I was a Fellow studying rheumatology. There were several receptionists who rotated the job with Margaret. It was a demanding and frustrating job. Except for Margaret, they all had a tendency to be irritable and unpleasant. Margaret was always pleasant, tolerant, understanding, and helpful. And she was the one with arthritis, severe deforming rheumatoid arthritis.

A year later, I was a Lahey Clinic Fellow at the New England Baptist Hospital, a much larger hospital next door to the Robert Breck Brigham, and the general hospital used by President Kennedy's family. The hospital lobby, a large cross-shaped space, had a reception area in the center with a counter enclosing three or four receptionists. Again, the most tolerant, kind, and thoughtful receptionist there was the woman with rheumatoid arthritis.

The emotional growth these women achieved helped them control their arthritis. Negative expectations, pessimism, hopelessness, and lack of control, are attitudes associated with impaired health. Socially isolated people develop more diseases and die sooner, while confident support and social involvement predict lower mortality.

Psychologists report that Brief Supportive-Expressive Group Therapy for women with metastatic breast cancer over a one-year period is associated with increased survival time. Positive meaning shifts are associated with better outcomes after a heart attack. HIV positive individuals who are more engaged with deep meaning life goals show better immune patterns. Supportive-Expressive Therapy employs a safe and supportive environment for patients to share similar traumas, victories, and defeats. It provides an opportunity for patients to help one another, to face and confront their fears, and to reorder their life priorities. A loving and caring spouse or companion can provide this kind of support.

Your immune cells, the lymphocytes, can't clone themselves as well if your mood is negative. Positive moods increase their ability to divide, multiply, and conquer. Negative moods depress the immune system and positive moods enhance it. Tests measuring the ability of lymphocytes to clone themselves and tests measuring levels of inflammatory cytokines document these immune changes. Loneliness, low attachment to a spouse, and poor marital quality are associated with immune system depression.

Stress and the endocrine system

Acute stress can have dramatic effects on arthritis. When I was drafted out of practice during the Viet Nam war, I had the good fortune to land at Walter Reed Army Medical Center in Washington, D.C. where I was responsible for the rheumatology clinic. Among the many fascinating experiences I enjoyed during my two years there, one involved the psychiatry department.

The psychiatrists in that department believed that they could predict exacerbations of rheumatoid arthritis and looked for a volunteer to help them test their theory. One retired man was willing to live in the hospital for a period of several months. During this time, blood tests were drawn more or less daily and 24 hour urine specimens were collected several times a week. (He is the only patient I've known who had so much blood drawn for tests that he became anemic and required a transfusion.) Meanwhile the psychiatrists interviewed him daily. One day they hit a hot spot involving personal issues between the volunteer and his parents. He became very upset, and his blood cortisol levels rose sharply. After a few days, when he became calm again, the cortisol levels dropped and his rheumatoid arthritis joint pain and swelling increased abruptly in a typical steroid-induced rebound phenomenon. We have known for decades that abrupt withdrawal of corticosteroids from a patient with rheumatoid arthritis will produce an acute flare of disease activity, but here the steroids weren't pills, but natural products of his endocrine system.

Acute stress stimulates the release of hormones from the pituitary gland at the base of the brain. This gland controls the production and release of corticosteroids and epinephrine. At the onset of acute stress two other important classes of hormones are released: endorphins and encephalins, the internal opioids. In addition to pain control, they act to block the release of LHRH, a hormone that controls ultimately the release of testosterone. Testosterone is responsible for the sex-drive in both men and women.

Endorphins, stress, and pain

The high one feels after exercising for about half an hour is from the effects of endorphins released from the pituitary gland, and encephalins mobilized mostly in the brain and spinal cord. The endorphins and encephalins shut off the pain fibers in the spinal cord. Many types of stress stimulate release of these internal opioids, including aerobic exercise, surgery, childbirth, cold exposure, and low blood sugar levels.

Acute stress produces protective responses; *chronic stress* depresses these responses. The chronic pain, function loss, and frustration of arthritis cause chronic stress. Chronic stress aggravates arthritis. Sex is an antidote. Some of the ways that sex has this kind of effect involve the interplay between the psyche and emotion, sexual arousal, oxytocin and prolactin from the endocrine system, and their effects on the immune system.

Oxytocin

Oxytocin is a hormone produced by the pituitary gland. It is best known as the hormone that induces labor and delivery in the birth of a baby and in signaling milk production. Long before that event, oxytocin plays a role when you first find that someone special. It is increased during sexual attraction both in women and in men. It increases during sexual excitement, peaks at orgasm and lingers before it wanes.

Prolactin

Prolactin is another hormone of the pituitary that is increased substantially after orgasm. This too, occurs in both women and men. This is the hormone that controls milk production and release. It rises to a peak at orgasm and remains elevated for more than 60 minutes afterward. Beyond its role in milk production and in the events surrounding orgasm, prolactin contributes significantly to the integrity of your immune system. If the pituitary gland is removed surgically, prolactin levels fall and with it the immune system fails too. Antibody production is reduced and the cell to cell response of the T cells is impaired. These immune functions are restored by prolactin administration. Prolactin administration in intact animals stimulates an increase in IL-2, which acts as a growth factor for activated T-Cells. It helps them clone. It also increases the activity of the NK natural killer cells.

PROLACTIN

- Promotes antibody production by B-lymphocytes.

- Promotes cloning of T-lymphocytes

- Has receptors on the cell walls of B and T lymphocytes.

- Is increased for more than 60 minutes after orgasm.

The role of other hormones

Other hormones lack the sexually stimulated changes exhibited by oxytocin and prolactin. Plasma concentrations of corticosteroids, FSH, progesterone, estrogen and beta-endorphin are unaffected by orgasm. There may be more to the beta-endorphin story though, as demonstrated by studies with naloxone which blocks the effects of opioids. Naloxone is a drug that blocks the receptors through which opioids such as morphine and the endorphins and encephalins work. The reduced response to painful stimuli caused by oxytocin is inhibited by naloxone. In animal studies, oxytocin has been proven to have a pain relieving effect. Naloxone blocks that analgesia. In addition to the pain relieving effect, oxytocin enhances (and naloxone reduces) the level of subjective arousal and pleasure at orgasm in humans. The effects of naloxone indicate that these must be opioid based effects. Yet efforts to document a release of endorphins during orgasm have not been fruitful. Could oxytocin itself have an opioid based pain relieving effect? Isn't this what you might expect of nature? Oxytocin plays a central role in labor and delivery of a baby, and right when you need it most, it is also a pain reliever. The effect of blocking opioid receptors with naloxone and its associated inhibition of sexual arousal and pleasure are certain evidence that endogenous opioids play a role in the human sexual response. In an animal study, oxytocin injections were repeated over a five-day period in both male and female animals. Pain decreased. Blood pressure also decreased 10 to 20 mm Hg, corticosteroid and insulin levels increased, and the healing rate of wounds increased.

OXYTOCIN

- Released during labor and delivery.

- Released during sexual attraction and orgasm.

- Relieves pain.

- Works like morphine and the endorphins

- Correlates with sexual pleasure and orgasmic intensity.

Exercise as stressor

Exercise is another example of a good stressor. Like sexual stimulation it too stimulates a release of prolactin, but unlike sex, it causes an increase in corticosteroids. Twenty women with rheumatoid arthritis participated in a one week program at a resort where they heard lectures on arthritis, participated in aquatic exercises and had a daily program of yoga, T'ai chi and meditation. They were tested both before and after the week at the resort. They felt better emotionally afterward. Tests demonstrated an increase in positive affect scores and a decrease in negative affect scores. They also reacted less vigorously to stress. Coping skills improved. These effects were associated with increases in blood levels of corticosteroids and prolactin and an increase in the ratio of corticosteroids to prolactin.

Frigidity

Pain, fear of pain, anxiety about the ability to satisfy the sexual partner, loss of sexual confidence, depression with the present and dread of the future, all may separately or together lead to impotence or frigidity.

Ann Hamilton had 12 years of experience in sexual counseling in a disabled living unit at an orthopedic hospital in England. She writes that sexual expression is likely to be limited in arthritis, even in those with the desire and the capacity to initiate or accept sexual activity. Arthritis in the hands limits the ability and reduces the desire to caress. Arthritis in the elbows and shoulders impairs the ability to embrace. Supporting one's own weight on the arms and shoulders becomes impossible. Hip, knee, or spinal arthritis limits the positions available for coitus. The necessity to avoid painful activities may interfere with the freedom of sexual expression.

Dryness (Sjogren's syndrome)

Dryness of the mucous membranes occurs with Sjogren's syndrome. This syndrome of dry eyes, dry mouth and dryness of other mucous membranes can accompany arthritis. It causes difficulty in kissing and in sexual intercourse due to the often profound dryness. There are medications that help, especially a recently introduced prescription medicine called Evoxac[R]. Associated dryness of the genitalia requires the use of lubricants.

Partner response

The sexual partner with a normal sexual drive in a normal body lacks the normal means of obtaining sexual satisfaction and release when the partner is unable to participate. They fear to cause pain or distress to their disabled partners. Both partners resent the restrictions that pain, fatigue, and reticence impose on their lovemaking. Spontaneity suffers.

A disabled woman feels guilty and inadequate because she is not behaving as she thinks a normal wife should. She is distressed about her diminished physical attractiveness. She fears her husband's rejection and desertion. The able-bodied husband may feel deprived and resentful of her behavior. When the arthritic partner is male, his ability to provide and his masculine role image suffer.

Loss of genital intercourse

A great deal of unnecessary distress is caused by the widely held concept among men that genital intercourse is the sole and ultimate aim of love and lovemaking. Then when genital intercourse is no longer possible or desirable, he ceases to express love to his partner. She feels a deep sense of loss and rejection. Correcting the approach, timing, and expectations of both partners can make for major improvements. Sharing thoughts, desires, and feelings with one another opens doors to healing. Both of the partners benefit emotionally and sexually.

A study by Muriel Shaul, "From early twinges to mastery: the process of adjustment in living with rheumatoid arthritis," looks at how women with rheumatoid arthritis experience their disease at different stages of their lives. Forty rheumatologists submitted referrals to the study to patients in their practices. From this group, women who participated in an annual telephone interview in 1989 and again in 1992 formed a group from which participants in this study were drawn. Participants were contacted, first by letter and then by telephone, to assess interest in participating in the study. They were then interviewed in person and asked to tell their story of rheumatoid arthritis. Thirty women were interviewed in their homes. Their average age was 54 years; 63% were married, and 37% were divorced, separated, or widowed.

A transition process with three stages was identified from the narratives. The first stage involved becoming aware of symptoms, and of the impact of symptoms on daily life. The second stage, learning to live with it, was an uneven and unpredictable process of trial and error, learning about the disease and life-management strategies. Most women in this study eventually achieved a "level of mastery" in which they managed everyday life in spite of the rheumatoid arthritis. Those who achieved a level of mastery managed not only the rheumatoid-arthritis-related symptoms, but also the associated role changes. They learned to use a variety of resources in managing the activities of daily life.

In the second stage, learning to live with arthritis, patients feared that their swelling and stiffness would persist and cause deformity. Fatigue added to the impact of reduced ability to function. Depression was prominent at this stage. The inability to carry out the duties of the patient's role in life as a mother, or provider, and as lover, added to the frustration and fatigue.

However, learning to live with the disease facilitated developing new techniques for getting things done and new interests to replace those that were no longer practical or possible. Then, finally goals and expectations were realigned and the patients reached a "mastery" stage.

Impediments to sex

The impediments of arthritis are similar to, but different from the impediments associated with aging. The greater incidence of osteoarthritis late in life combines the two for most of us. The effects of aging on sexuality call to mind the story of a man whose friend decided to send him a very special birthday gift to celebrate his 90th birthday. On the appointed day, the doorbell rang and there stood a gorgeous, naked young woman.

> "What can I do for you?" he asked.
>
> "Well, I'm here to give you super sex," she replied sweetly.
>
> The man thought for a minute and said, "I guess I'll take the soup."

Partners with arthritis have many of the same circumstances as the older patient. Desire persists, but the ability to perform has decreased in a variety of different ways. Usually younger people have the capacity for sexual responsiveness, even if it's impaired. If there is an altered self-image, foreplay and afterplay become all the more important. Gentle caressing, hugging, and expressions of affection are more significant here than anywhere else.

If a couple has lost interest in sex, and especially if this is due to the impact of arthritis, it can be awakened again. Subtle hints may be nothing more than a beginning. Remember the things that piqued your partner's interest in earlier days, and try again.

My perspective

People respond in several ways upon learning that they have arthritis, but often the expression of grief—from denial to anger to depression—intrudes on their process of mastering the disease. Eventually they learn to live with it, and our new medicines make it much easier. For those with residual damage from arthritis, mastering the disease can be accomplished by deciding not to give their lives over to the disease, and instead develop new, more easily achievable interests, and find ways to accomplish what they choose to accomplish. Attitude is tremendously important. People who have mastered their arthritis tend to be the most wonderful, kind, understanding, and considerate people.

Advice from a woman who "mastered" arthritis 47 years ago: Mastering arthritis can be done in small ways, like choosing to wash dishes by hand rather than using an automatic dishwasher, because movement of the hands in hot water helps to keep hands supple. Or walk the three blocks to the library instead of driving, because the walk is good exercise, and sunshine imparts vitamin D and lifts the spirits. As far as full body exercise in warm water: why not have sex in the swimming pool at night, after the neighbors go to bed? And don't forget your sense of humor.

Remember the importance of support. Both partners need to remember that, and to work on their partnership. Those who have a supportive relationship, and who are socially involved, also have a happier existence and reduced morbidity and mortality. Love one another.

7

Quackery and Fraud

In 1901, just over a hundred years ago, President Teddy Roosevelt sent American troops to the Philippines to control the Muslim terrorists operating there. At that time, willow bark tea was the major remedy for arthritis. Scientists extracted the active ingredient in that tea, purified, analyzed, and synthesized it, and finally marketed it in 1901 as Bayer Aspirin.

That was the first of our modern medicines for arthritis. Since then, the volumes we've learned about the disease of arthritis and its treatment have made a huge difference in the quality of life for arthritis patients. Unfortunately, Muslim terrorists are still a problem in the Philippines.

It was also during the presidency of Teddy Roosevelt that the U.S. Congress wrote and passed the Pure Food and Drug Act of 1906, taking aim at fraudulent practices and quackery.

Safety and The Pure Food and Drug Act.

Subsequent to the passing of the Pure Food and Drug Act by the U.S. Congress, all drugs (allopathy) of Western medicine must have a scientifically demonstrated effectiveness and safety before they may be marketed. At least that is the ideal. Complementary and alternative therapies, consisting of a broad range of physical, herbal, dietary, and psychological applications to treating disease and promoting health (including naturopathy, traditional folk medicine, and even simple fraud), operate under a different standard. These therapies and drugs are marketed without proof of effectiveness or safety. Any existing loopholes in the law (designed and set in place to protect the American public) are hastily manipulated by marketers whose health products and foods are advertised and sold as effective.

Some alternatives are based on valid and valuable herbal medicines that date from early hunter-gatherer societies. Many of these have known pharmacological functions, and others contain less well-identified pharmacologically active compounds. Some alternatives however, are intentional quackery.

Quacks promote questionable cures that may involve special metals, or energies, or natural things like food, herbs, or water, or mechanical things that can shake, rattle, and roll you to better health. The U.S. government estimates that Americans spend $10 billion a year on worthless remedies.

According to the *Oxford English Dictionary*, the word "quack," or "quackery," is a mid 17th century abbreviation of a Dutch word, "quacksalver", which is probably from the obsolete "quacken", or "prattle" + "salf", (meaning "salve"). Put it all together and we have prattlers about salve, or fast-talking salesmen of questionable medicines.

However, it seems the practice of quackery dates back even further, since the Oath of Hippocrates dates from

500 BC. The Oath enjoins physicians to commit to following a treatment regimen for the benefit of the patient and abstain from deleterious and mischievous cures.

The Hippocratic Oath

One of the ceremonies involved in graduation from medical school is the administration of the Hippocratic Oath. Considering that this oath has been handed down for more than 2000 years, you may find it both interesting and remarkably contemporary.

The Oath of Hippocrates

> *I swear by Apollo the physician, and AEsculapius, and Health, and All-heal, and all the gods and goddesses, that, according to my ability and judgment, I will keep this oath and this stipulation—to reckon him who taught me this Art equally dear to me as my parents, to share my substance with him and relieve his necessities if required; to look upon his offspring in the same footing as my own brothers, and to teach them this Art, if they shall wish to learn it, without fee or stipulation; and that by precept, lecture, and every other mode of instruction, I will impart a knowledge of the Art to my own sons, and those of my teachers, and to disciples bound by a stipulation and oath according to the law of medicine, but to none others.*

> *I will follow that system of regimen which, according to my ability and judgment, I consider for the benefit of my patients, and abstain from whatever is deleterious and mischievous.*

I will give no deadly medicine to any one if asked, nor suggest any such counsel; and in like manner I will not give to a woman a pessary to produce an abortion.

With purity and with holiness I will pass my life and practice my Art. I will not cut persons laboring under the stone, but will leave this to be done by men who are practitioners of this work.

Into whatever houses I enter, I will go into them for the benefit of the sick, and will abstain from every voluntary act of mischief and corruption; and, further, from the seduction of females or males, of freemen and slaves.

Whatever, in connection with my professional practice or not in connection with it, I see or hear, in the life of men, which ought not to be spoken of abroad, I will not divulge, as reckoning that all such should be kept secret.

While I continue to keep this Oath unviolated, may it be granted to me to enjoy life and the practice of the Art, respected by all men, in all times! But should I trespass and violate this Oath, may the reverse be my lot!

Illusions, delusions, and lies

Some quacks are charlatans, the con artists who know that their cures don't work. These crooks lie about their credentials and fabricate success stories. Polished, persuasive, smooth talkers, they con people into paying for their fake cures. America's celebrated showman, P. T. Barnum, launched his career by writing advertisement for a baldness cure. He's also the one who said, "There's a sucker born every minute."

Some quacks are only wishful thinkers. These are the delusional quacks who are convinced without proof that their impossible product works. But wishful thinkers exist on both sides of the sale. The seller may have a poor understanding of scientific principles and may truly believe that their remedies work. They often claim that modern science hasn't yet been able to prove that these remedies work. Buyers become wishful thinkers when they use unproved remedies. They wish it to be so, therefore they think it is so, therefore they conclude that it is. Wishful thinking flows from impatience and drives these buyers to determine that if medical science can't cure them, then they will go find their own cure. But what they find is too often nothing more than a hoax. One amusing example is soil that the promoters claimed was gathered on the moon and returned to the U.S. by astronauts.

Moondust

Moon dust was a secret. Soil samples brought back to Earth from the moon were kept secret and secure by the federal government. Somehow the promoter was able to acquire, or pretend to acquire, a supply large enough to market. Buyers, they claimed, would have their arthritis cured.

Earthdust

Dust from the earth, or more precisely, dirt, has been processed into capsule form and sold as medicine. Not many years ago, two clinics operating near the U.S.-Mexican border were found to be treating Americans who sought a cure for their arthritis. These people lined up for hours, passed through the "clinic," received no examination, and were passed on to purchase the "prescribed medications," on the way out. These medications consisted of a variety of tablets and capsules.

The patients took these medications, felt better, and believed that their arthritis was getting better.

U.S. clinical laboratories analyzed these medications discovering that despite the clinic's claims that there was no prednisone or cortisone in the capsules, there was, and that is why patients felt better. Another ingredient was a tranquilizer (typically Valium, an anti-anxiety drug) which provided nothing more than a short-term relief from the anxiety that usually accompanies any illness. The rest of the pills, analyzed and reanalyzed for confirmation, contained nothing but dirt, soil, and "earthdust".

Several of my patients went to Mexico to get some of that "medication," and developed serious complications from the prednisone. They reported that the doctor at the Mexican clinic, if he was a doctor, told them that there was no prednisone or cortisone in the prescribed pills. When the medication ran out, their arthritis symptoms and pain, inadequately controlled worsened, and came back in full force.

Water

One company sold a product that they claimed is able to concentrate water. A dose of this special water additive was to be added to a gallon of distilled water And they claimed that the treated water increases the rate of chemical reactions, neutralizes excess acid and alkaline solutions in the body, acts as a penetrant, and picks up and carries unwanted or toxic substances which then the body excretes.

They said that the water is energized or activated, and that it becomes thinner, wetter, and "polymerized", and that this allows it to more easily penetrate the surface of all the estimated 13 trillion cells of the body. But the fact is that you can't polymerize water and if you did it would make the molecule and the resulting material thicker, denser, less wet, and less able to penetrate the surface of cells, just the opposite of the huckster's claim. Polymerization means the hooking together of many molecules of the chemical being polymerized. Typically, the process of polymerization begins with a liquid solution of a single kind of molecule, and after adding a tiny amount of an enzyme it becomes polymerized; it becomes a solid. Plastics are made this way. Sugar is another example. Starting with a solution of sugar in water, an enzyme is added and this causes the sugar molecules to polymerize, or hook together in very long chains. The sugar thus becomes cellulose, wood. Termites have an enzyme that lets them break down the cellulose of wood into sugar molecules, depolymerization. Thus, they can digest wood.

The hucksters also claimed that their special water claws or grabs at nutrients and then more readily opens the doors to cell walls, allowing it to deliver the nutrients into the cell. Since it also assists in removal of the waste products from the cell, cellular nutrition is enhanced. It improves digestion and reduces the necessary volume of food intake and nutritional supplements. And of course it must therefore also benefit the immune system. They also say that it improves digestion in ileostomy patients and in horses. They describe the experience of one couple who were raising Arabian horses and were able to cut grain from 12 pounds per day for each horse to 4 pounds per day, because the horses were nourished on so much less food. Added to this, the con artists say, is the fact that many *humans* can reduce their meals from 3 per day to one, reduce the nutritional supplements from one half to one third, and reap major benefits to the immune system! This is all pseudoscientific double-talk!

Before I would spend a nickel on a product like this, or recommend it to my patients, I would have to see the science. When something smells fishy, generally there is a fish around somewhere.

Radon water

Specially treated water has been invoked as a cure in a number of claims. One of these claims reads: "Drink your way to health and happiness with a special water jug in your home. Just fill the jug at night. The water remains in contact with the radium-ore walls for twelve hours. By morning the water has returned to that healthful state found only at the springs." This is one of those cases where I smell fish, but read on.

Radon spas

Radon produces low-level radiation, which for years has been credited with arthritis relief. The concept, called "hormesis", states that low levels of an inert gas, Radon-222 (a naturally occurring product of the radio-active decay of uranium) may be beneficial, even though high doses are harmful. Radon "spas" are an accepted part of health care in Eastern Europe and Japan. They include Gasteiner Heilstollen in Austria, Fuerstenzeche "Duke's Mine" in Germany, the Radium Palace in the Czech Republic, and the radon spa at Misawa, Japan, and many others.

The "radon for health" phenomenon in the United States began in 1951 when the wife of a mining engineer discovered that her bursitis improved dramatically after visiting the Free Enterprise mine in Montana. Barbra Erickson, an anthropology doctoral candidate at the University of Nevada, has written in detail about this phenomenon and was kind enough to let me share it with you here.

> *"Tucked away in the Elkhorn Mountains of Montana, about halfway between the cities of Butte and Helena, are six small and obscure mines, doing their best to make a living by attracting visitors. Old mines like these, no longer worked for their*

A sign in downtown Boulder directs the would-be visitor to turn onto a side street, which quickly becomes gravel. The road passes under the interstate, which has so little traffic on it that it seems like a deserted bridge and winds uphill for two miles past sagebrush and the occasional cow. The Free Enterprise building sits on the top of a small hill, surrounded by a parking lot, and a row of RV hookups... Part of the attraction of the place is the quietness, as well as the sage- and evergreen-scented breeze that always seems to be blowing. A person can imagine feeling healed here.

In addition to the Free Enterprise mine, which was the first, other "spa" mines in the area include the Merry Widow, Earth Angel, High Ore, Sunshine, and Lone Tree Mines.

Anecdotes describe the reported responses of visitors to the mines. These are not scientifically controlled observations and they are subject to psychological and emotionally based responses. Nonetheless, they are the reasons why people believe in the mines.

One man described a woman he saw when she first arrived at the radon mines:

> 'She'd been completely bed-ridden—all her joints were just frozen up. She was always in pain, and said she just felt hopeless and depressed. Her husband had to carry her from her bed to the couch to the bathroom. But when they left she was walking! ...and now they come every year.'

Ronald, a mine visitor of 63, described his Ankylosing Spondylitis as a 'disease which fuses the bones of the back together.' He says when he first came to the mine in

1987, he could hardly walk, but after four series of treatments, two and three years apart, he no longer uses a cane, and says that his doctor considers him to be 'a walking miracle.'

Can these and other anecdotal cures be attributed to a placebo effect? Possibly, but the attitude of the patients who related the stories reflects a willingness to believe in the cure, regardless of the true cause:

> '...And of course people say it's all in your head. And I say, well if it is, good! If you can believe that you're not sick and you don't even have to take medication, so what? At least there's no side effects, it's all in your head.'

> And 'We've had dogs go down there [into the mine] with arthritis, and the dogs went running around after that—if it's the placebo effect, well then, who told the dog?'"

Concerns about radiation exposure are worrisome. However the number and stature of the scientists, including M.D.s and Ph.D.s from leadership positions in prestigious institutions who say that low-dose radon is safe and actually beneficial is reassuring.

A red light in a box

Even a simple red light in a black box has been used to represent a therapeutic machine. For a fee, patients would insert their hands into the machine for arthritis treatment.

Another red-light-in-a-box cure included what was described as a "special kind of red light". This battery operated, pocket-sized gadget was claimed to activate cell DNA to produce an abundance of protein and calcium, and accelerate tissue healing. A long and complex description of how and why this red light was therapeutic used pseudo-scientific double talk to deceive. It was claimed to be totally harmless, free of side effects, and could provide a long list of therapeutic benefits, including pain relief, arthritis relief, muscle relaxation, ulcer and wound healing, cure of asthma, headaches, skin conditions and food allergies, etc.

Pulsators, shakers, and vibrators

The "Macaura Pulsocon" was created and promoted by Gerald Macaura. This self-proclaimed "vibrotherapist" founded an institute in Manchester, England in 1908 that featured drugless cures. One of the devices he created was the Pulsator, later called the Pulsocon. It was a hand-held device that looked like an eggbeater. As it was held against the skin, the wheel would turn, and the skin felt vibration. It was claimed to increase circulation, loosen joints, and eliminate chronic pain. Macaura rented theaters and staged some very popularly attended lectures to advertise this device. He left England in 1911 to work in continental Europe, and found himself expelled from Prussia in 1912 for an "attempt to cheat." In Paris, he was sentenced and fined for swindling and practicing medicine illegally. At the same time, the Cirkulon Institute of Kansas City, Missouri, distributed this same device under the brand name "Cirkulon" for $15.

The "Vibrometer" was used for applying massage by vibratory motion. This device used a small motor powered wheel with tacks to pluck the strings of a banjo-like instrument. It was said to cure ailments by musical vibrations.

And the "Battle Creek Combination Vibratory Chair" was claimed to be four machines in one: a vibrating chair, a vibrating footstool, a vibrating bar, and a foot vibrator. It vibrated vigorously and a treatment lasting three to five minutes and claimed to do many beneficial things, such as relaxing muscles, relieving pain, improving circulation, respiration, metabolism and excretion.

Magnets

Magnets for arthritis have been featured items for a long time. Magnetized copper bracelets are claimed to relieve arthritis, neuritis, and general soreness. Other variations include magnetic bandages, belts, caps, leggings, lung protectors, mattresses, patches, shoe insoles, and even a magnetic throat shield to prevent colds. Magnets have been promoted on the theory that they make people healthier by improving their connection to the earth's magnetic field, aligning the elements in the human body, increasing blood flow, blocking pain signals, altering the acid/alkaline balance of bodily fluids, attracting the iron in the blood and changing the migration of calcium ions in the body to heal broken bones and remove calcium from arthritis joints. None of these theories are consistent with known scientific principles.

Magnetic forces can affect bone growth. Imagine a laboratory setting, where a bone that is placed in an apparatus to hold it steady, receives a force applied to the side of the bone, halfway between the ends of the bone. This activity stimulates bone growth on the side opposite to the applied force. The bone on the same side as the source of force gets reabsorbed. The balance between new bone formation and reabsorption of previously formed bone is largely controlled by mechanical strain.

In this same environment, negative electrical charges occur on the side opposite the force or tension, while positive charges occur on the same side as the tension. Electrons migrate to the compressed side, creating a negative charge that disappears if the compression is maintained. As compression is released, an equal and opposite positive pulse appears as the electrons bounce back into place. Hydroxyapatite and collagen are the components of bone that participate in this phenomenon. When they are deformed, it creates an electric potential. The idea of using magnets or TENS Transcutaneous Electrical Nerve Stimulation (See below) units to create the electrical potentials desired for healing is based on these observations.

This also explains the merits of weight bearing exercise to preserve bone density. Stresses applied to bone produce the electrical potentials that stimulate new bone formation. Cartilage integrity is similarly affected. The electrical potential stimulates bone and cartilage growth.

The effectiveness of magnets for arthritis remains dubious in the face of limited research, however pulsed electro-magnetic fields are useful in fracture healing, and potential clinical applications for osteoarthritis, osteoporosis, and wound healing do exist. The possibility that magnets might help to provide temporary relief of pain prompted the marketing of magnets for patients to self-treat. So far, the benefits appear to be merely financial, and in favor of the marketer. Patients appear to benefit chiefly by the placebo effect.

TENS

Transcutaneous Electrical Nerve Stimulation (TENS) is used to reduce pain by sending subliminal pain signals to the brain. The process is accomplished by providing a low voltage electrical stimulus that causes a sensory signal. This signal runs to the spinal cord and interferes with chronic pain signals typical of low back syndromes. TENS has also been tested in ankylosing spondylitis, a rheumatoid variant that involves the low back. The method provided significant differences in pain and stiffness compared to sham TENS treated controls.

Many patients with fibromyalgia have felt relief after receiving TENS treatments. In this situation, the chronic pain signals and their subsequent exaggeration by the central nervous system are the major element of the disease. TENS can help modulate pain perception, but it hasn't been effective enough.

One study showed that TENS was marginally helpful either alone, or with electroacupuncture and ice massage in patients with osteoarthritis of the knee. In a double blind, randomized, placebo controlled study conducted by a consortium of research centers, pulsed electrical stimulation (TENS) was delivered at night for four weeks. Dr. Zizic and colleagues reported that it produced significant short-term improvement in knee pain, function, movement and stiffness in their patients with osteoarthritis of the knee.

8

Herbal, Mineral and Homeopathic Remedies

> *"It is a capital mistake to theorize before one has data. Insensibly, one begins to twist facts to suit theories, instead of theories to suit fact."*
>
> Sir Arthur Conan Doyle, *A Scandal in Bohemia*

Medicine shows were popular in the mid-1800s, especially in rural areas where there wasn't much entertainment. Salesmen barnstormed around the country selling nostrums like Kickapoo, Indian Sagwa, and Magic Wizard Oil. Today we group their products together and call them snake oil.

These medicine shows followed a typical pattern. First, an opening act that consisted of a magic act or comedy routine was used to get the crowd into a happy and receptive mood. Next, the salesman would describe frightening stories of regular people who had fallen from good health into serious illness, such as arthritis, tuberculosis, or cancer. Then of course, the salesman would offer hope and redemption through his products. Part of this pitch included a demonstration of the effectiveness of the product, using it on a hired actor or someone from the audience (either a plant or a gullible local).

Medicine Show Slang

The medicine show trade even developed its own slang, revealing the true perspective of these salesmen.

- **Lot Lice** - people who came to the show but didn't buy anything
- **Herbal Medicine** - chopped grass
- **Bally Act** - an added attraction, like dancing girls
- **Alagazam** - the pitchman's hello
- **Velvet** – profit

Medicine shows were cited in a civil movement that led to the passage of the Pure Food and Drug Act of 1906. Then as now, people bought false hopes.

Homeopathy and the history of U.S. pharmaceutical regulation

Largely due to the efforts of Royal Copeland, a U.S. Senator from New York, the 1938 Food, Drug, and Cosmetic act recognized homeopathic pharmacopoeia as drugs without requiring proof of effectiveness and safety. These substances were simply "grandfathered" in, under cover and into public use. Senator Copeland was a prominent homeopathic physician. Since safety was the primary consideration at the time, and the extreme dilution of homeopathic remedies made them seem innocuous, Congress permitted these products to be exempted from restriction.

In 1962, the Kefauver-Harris Amendment was passed. It was designed to require that all drugs had to be proved effective and safe before they could be marketed. A legal battle was on the horizon and homeopathic remedies were in danger of exclusion. The Food and Drug Administration didn't press the issue, and this allowed over-the-counter remedies to escape the requirement for proof of effectiveness and safety. If you read the advertisements for over-the-counter health promotions closely, you will see the caveat, printed there by law, that the product, though offered to relieve some condition or illness, "is not promoted for the diagnosis or treatment of any disease."

Samuel Christian Hahnemann was a German physician and theorist who lived in the era preceding the growth of scientific knowledge. He was the first to propose that a sick person could be cured if given minute doses of a substance that caused the same symptoms in a healthy person. He called this "the law of similia," or similars. His method was called homeopathy, from the Greek words homios (like) and pathos (suffering). The combination of the "law of similia" with another pronouncement of Hahnemann, "the law of infinitesimals" makes up the essence of homeopathic pharmacy.

In "the law of infinitesimals," he argued that the more diluted the dose, the more powerful the remedy. This sounds just like the definition of an expert: someone who knows more and more about less and less, until he knows everything about nothing. In a variable but basic homeopathic tradition, one drop of the active ingredient is diluted 30 times, then one drop of the 30:1 dilution is diluted 30 times, and this is repeated for 30 30:1 dilutions. Nothing is left, so the toxic material that started the dilution is no longer toxic, but in its emptiness, it is inert. There is none of it left. You are buying nothing.

Meanwhile, the over-the counter remedies remain unregulated, unproved, and unsound, thanks to the influence of Senator Royal Copeland, the homeopath. The tendency of the uneducated to succumb to the promotions of quacks is understandable. This has been our history since the time of Hippocrates. But today, with a highly educated populace and broad understanding of scientifically proven fact, why do we spend $10 billion a year in the U.S. alone for unproven remedies? We are wishful thinkers who don't think.

Are natural products healthier?

Natural substances include strychnine, lead, arsenic, and mercury. A natural substance typically consists of many components. Synthesizing a compound requires molecular isolation of a pure compound.

In his book, *Quacks, Fakers, and Charlatans in English Medicine*, Roy Porter published a telling image depicting a drunken satyr cavorting atop the globe. On the right are physicians and quacks fighting for legitimacy, and on the left stands a blindfolded justice with scales tipped by a lawyer's money. This image dates from about 1800, and its significance remains today as an allegory of a world of justice and health turned over into one of chance and greed.

DHEA (dehydroepiandrosterone)

DHEA is a weak male hormone (steroid) produced by the adrenal glands that is converted into testosterone. In rheumatoid arthritis and lupus, its presence is reduced. It is important in up-regulating the production of the cytokine Interleukin-2 in normal T-cells. When administered to mice with murine lupus, a dramatic reverse in their clinical autoimmune disease is seen. Giltay et al conducted the first reported uncontrolled trial in patients with active rheumatoid arthritis. The study report stated that none of the efficacy variables changed significantly. In another study, "DHEA as adjunctive therapy for patients with lupus", was associated with a significant decrease in disease activity. It remains a subject of scientific interest and ongoing investigation.

DHEA is not risk-free. First, since it converts to testosterone in the body, it can lead to prostate enlargement in men and masculinization in women. Second, it is associated with potential risk of liver damage, heart disease, insulin resistance, and promotion of uterine, ovarian, and breast cancers. Some naturopaths and physicians versed in naturopathy recommend use of DHEA, and some don't.

Chaparral

Chaparral is an herbal preparation made from the desert shrub of the same name, and is commonly used for its antioxidant properties. A report by D. W. Gordon, et al, in the February 8, 1995 issue of the *Journal of the American Medical Association*, discussed a 60-year-old woman who took chaparral. After taking chaparral for 10 months, this woman developed severe hepatitis and ultimately required a liver transplant. She recovered after the transplant, but the concern that chaparral could cause serious liver injury raised alarm.

Currently chaparral is hard to find in stores and on the Internet. However, I found it on one site, and the claims for its amazing capacities read like prototypical quackery, including no warning about the danger involved in consuming this shrub and it's derivatives.

There is a soundly reasoned concern among healthcare professionals that nutriceuticals (which increase in popularity yearly), have the power to cause significant toxicity and/or drug interactions. Of course there is a long history of nutriceuticals being used medicinally among nature-based cultures, a practice that has existed far beyond the history of Western medicine. However, in those cultures, elders trained apprentice practitioners in their healing craft, and the practitioners treated patients.

While there are highly trained and knowledgeable naturopaths treating many people in our culture today, more people go into health food stores and take their advice from clerks behind the counter who barely know how to run the cash register. They trust their health to faith in nature. While there are exceptions, most of what they take has not been tested for safety or effectiveness, and is sold without oversight, review, or approval by regulatory agencies. Law prohibits sellers from marketing these substances as diagnostics or disease treatment, so while the sellers deny that the products are marketed for treatment, they wink at the obvious and continue to promote and sell their products with the intent to treat.

Ginger

> *"He walks again!! Ancient spice cures famous film star crippled by arthritis. Within short months of adding this venerable herb to his diet, this aged man is running marathons again."*

I'll admit that I'm exaggerating the glossy brochure that patient after patient brought into my office to show me, but it disturbs me every time I think about it. It's not that the author of the promotional shouting was wrong about using the spice for arthritis, but the information isn't new! It had only been forgotten by enough people to make it seem new. It is flat out dishonest to promote something very old as a breakthrough.

Ginger is, as you know, an East Indian cooking spice scientifically known as *Zingiber officinale*. Interestingly, it is described in ancient Ayurvedic and Tibb traditional East Indian healing systems of medicine as useful in rheumatism or inflammation. Often there are naturally occurring therapeutic agents in natural remedies. In the case of ginger, a literature review reveals several current articles that discuss the effects of this popular ancient remedy. In November 2001, R.D. Altman, M.D. and K.C. Marcussen, published a related study in the prominent rheumatology journal *Arthritis and Rheumatism.* The report, "Effects of a ginger extract on knee pain in patients with osteoarthritis," described a study of 261 patients with osteoarthritis of the knee. Participation in this double blind study that compared ginger to a placebo, required that patients have moderate to severe knee pain.

The study was performed simultaneously throughout several medical centers cooperating under the same protocol. Using several different clinics is preferred because it reduces the risk of accidental bias that a skewed result from one clinic can produce. The six-week treatment, using a highly purified and standardized ginger extract, found that it had a moderate but significant effect on reducing symptoms of osteoarthritis of the knee. Side effects consisted mostly of mild gastrointestinal irritation.

Another relevant study, "A randomized, placebo-controlled cross-over study of ginger extracts and ibuprofen in osteoarthritis," was reported from the Parker Institute Department of Rheumatology in Frederiksburg Hospital, Copenhagen, Denmark. In this double blind, crossover study, ginger extract was compared to a placebo and ibuprofen in patients with osteoarthritis of the hip or knee. To eliminate carry-over effects from previous medications, patients went without medication for a "washout" period of one week prior to the study, followed by three segments of three weeks on each treatment: ginger, ibuprofen, and placebo. The three treatments followed a randomized sequence to avoid a pattern of one treatment preceding and influencing another.

Symptoms were measured with an index of disease activity called the Lequesne index, a standardized interview system that assigns scores for pain at night, after immobilization, while standing, walking, and on getting up after sitting. It also assigns up to six points for decreasing ability to walk, movement limitations such as climbing or descending stairs, squatting, and walking on uneven ground. Added to these parameters is the investigator's judgment of effectiveness of the treatment under double blind conditions at the end of the study.

By ranking the effectiveness of the three treatment periods in the first three week segment of the study, ibuprofen was shown to be more effective than ginger extract, and ginger was better than placebo in reducing pain and improving symptoms. No significant difference in effectiveness could be seen between placebo, ibuprofen, and ginger extract during the second and third segments of the study. There were no serious adverse events with ginger or ibuprofen. The authors concluded that the study showed a statistically significant effect of ginger extract only during the first period of the study, and only with explorative statistical methods. In other words, the effectiveness of ginger was open to interpretation.

In yet another study, severe arthritis was induced in the right knee and right paw of male rats by injecting them with a material called Freund's adjuvant. Freund's adjuvant is a substance made of killed microorganisms (mycobacteria) in an oil and water emulsion that is administered to induce development of a particular type of inflammation. As treatment, Eugenol (a material made from clove oil with analgesic properties) and ginger oil were each given orally to different groups of rats for 26 days. Both oils caused a significant suppression of paw and joint swelling. This study suggested that both eugenol and ginger oil have potent anti-inflammatory and antirheumatic properties.

Powdered ginger was used to treat 56 patients, including 28 with rheumatoid arthritis, 18 with osteoarthritis, and 10 with muscular discomfort unrelated to arthritis. More than three quarters of these arthritis patients experienced varying degrees of relief from pain and swelling. All of the patients with muscular discomfort (as separate from arthritis) experienced relief from pain. None of the patients reported adverse effects while they were taking ginger for periods ranging from three months to two and a half years.

Herbal medicines receive attention by authentic scientists. When technology allows further efforts, they are re-examined. It is important to realize that anything that has potential to be significantly effective in arthritis is going to be studied, extracted, patented, and marketed by our sophisticated pharmaceutical industry. They are unlikely to miss anything because of the profit potential. However, it's wiser to wait for careful studies to document both safety and effectiveness before challenging our bodies with unproved remedies.

Ginseng

Ubiquitous ginseng is another example of a nutriceutical that has received substantial interest since antiquity, and it's a focus of interest again now. In Korea the rice paddies are rimmed by a row of taller shrubs, which are ginseng plants. Six-packs of bottles similar to soft drink bottles, each holding a ginseng root in a golden solution, are sold everywhere in Korea. While visiting, I decided I would buy a single bottle for a souvenir. The saleslady was aghast that I wanted only one bottle. I still have it. One of my patients gave me a pack of ginseng cigarettes. And soft drinks containing ginseng are currently popular and available throughout the United States.

Dr. J.Y. Cho is an M.D. who worked in the department of immunopharmacology at the Research and Development Center of the Dae Woong Pharmaceutical Company,

Sungnam, Korea. He reported data that suggest that these ginseng compounds possess potential therapeutic effectiveness against TNF-alpha mediated disease (which is a brief description of rheumatoid arthritis). He said also that the therapeutic potency of these agents may be enhanced when combined with various other TNF-alpha antagonists, further substantiating their role in blocking the effects of TNF alpha.

This is an example of the interest shown by a modern pharmaceutical company in investigating the potential utility of an old herbal remedy. They used appropriate scientific methods and published their findings in a legitimate peer-reviewed scientific journal. There is significant oversight and review by objective and unassociated experts in this kind of research publication. Unlike the glossy advertising and hoopla dependant on testimonies by individuals who may be misled or who may be swayed by personal gain, this scientific approach is far more believable.

Another report, "The anti-inflammatory activity of ginsenoside RO," by H. Matsuda and associates, was published in *Planta Med* in 1990. It describes a study in which this ginsenoside RO component of ginseng inhibited an acute swelling of the rat paw which had been induced by injecting Compound 48-80, or carrageenin. This report, of course, points to the possibility of relief from arthritis-swollen joints.

Ginko Biloba

Another example of alternative medicine used for arthritis includes ginkgo biloba, and studies have demonstrated possible benefits in animals. In humans, its use is predominantly for mental acuity and to retard memory loss by increasing circulation. No studies have documented effectiveness against arthritis in humans.

Noni juice

Noni juice has recently been advertised heavily and with glowing claims. Morinda citrifolia, or Noni, has been used in Polynesian folk medicine for over 2000 years. It is known as Indian Mulberry in India, ba ji tian in China, nono in Tahiti, and noni in Hawaii. The fruit juice of this plant contains a polysaccharide rich component that can be precipitated out. Noni-precipitate or noni-ppt has been studied and is believed to have anti-inflammatory, anti-histamine, anti-bacterial, anti-viral, anti-fungal, anti-cancer, hypotensive, and pain relieving effects.

Is this too good to be true? One study by Hirazumi and Furusawa described Noni's anti-tumor activity in mice. It improved survival time and had "curative effects" when it was combined with sub-optimal doses of the standard chemotherapeutic agents, adriamycin, cisplatin, 5-fluorouracil, and vincristine. Many studies have suggested anti-cancer effects, but none are conclusive.

Noni also is capable of stimulating the release of several immune mediators including the cytokines TNF-alpha, interleukin-1-beta, interleukin-10, interleukin 12p70 and interferon-gamma. It suppresses interleukin-4 release but has no effect on interleukin-2. It also stimulates the generation of nitric oxide which is destructive and contributes to joint tissue damage. TNF-alpha and interleukin 1 are two of the most destructive elements in rheumatoid arthritis. Therefore, Noni is capable of making arthritis worse.

Several studies document noni's ability to scavenge superoxide radicals. This suggests a mechanism that would allow it to be useful in arthritis and many other conditions, but there have been no studies that demonstrated effectiveness against arthritis.

Other herbs

Of the many herbs that have been used and promoted for arthritis, those named above are examples of some for which we have some reliable information. The Arthritis Foundation is a reliable source of substantial information about herbs for arthritis, and you may contact them by calling their regional office in the large city nearest to your home (or www.arthritis.org). The PDR for Herbal Medicines is another book that is an excellent source of information.

Minerals, trace elements

Recorded history dating to ancient Egypt in 1550 BCE documents the use of trace elements, especially those containing metallic compounds for treating musculoskeletal disorders. Today, we know that they are metabolically important in processes involving collagen, bone, and the immune system. They are components of enzymes, including those that inactivate reactive oxygen molecules, so important in inflammation and tissue destruction. Their physiological role is substantial. Are they useful therapeutically? That is not so certain.

Copper

The use of copper salts as therapeutic agents was first recorded in the Ebers papyrus dating from 1550 BC. Arthritis patients have worn copper amulets, anklets, and bracelets for thousands of years, but there are no good studies to support any substantial anti-arthritic effects. Using questionnaires and psychological parameters as outcome measures, one poorly controlled trial suggested some therapeutic value in copper bracelets, hypothesizing that copper was systemically absorbed since it is soluble in human sweat.

Copper bracelets remain popular, but are an unfounded alternative treatment for arthritis. According to one concept, if you wear a copper bracelet that fits around the wrist with a gap between the two ends, electrons jump across the gap, which somehow cures your arthritis.

I recall, when I was an intern at San Francisco's Saint Mary's Hospital, I saw a 90-year-old patient who was admitted to the hospital for investigation of an undiagnosed illness. I noticed that he wore a copper wire around his left ankle, and asked him why he wore it. "Well, Doc. I can't remember why I put it on, but I'm afeared to take it off."

Many patients and even some rheumatologists wear copper bracelets; some in hope, some in curiosity, and some just for fun. Whatever the reason, the thought has occurred to me that maybe the Arthritis Foundation should capitalize on the copper bracelet craze as a moneymaking project. There's certainly a market for them. As a fundraiser for research into the causes and cure of arthritis, the Foundation could market bracelets with the Foundation logo and a disclaimer, "Wear a copper bracelet. It won't cure your arthritis, but it will help us find a cure." When I suggested this to the Foundation's Northern California Chapter, it was rejected because they feared people would be misled into thinking the bracelet had curative effects.

Selenium

This trace mineral is said to have anti-inflammatory effects. Selenium levels were found to be lower in a group of 87 patients with rheumatoid arthritis compared to normal controls. Greater reductions were noted in patients with the most severe disease. In a double-blind placebo controlled trial, selenium in a dose of 200 mcg daily was associated with reduction of joint pain and inflammation in six of eight women, while there was no change in the placebo group. Selenium was ineffective in another study.

Zinc

The purported anti-inflammatory effect of zinc prompted a study in 24 refractory (stubborn) chronic rheumatoid arthritis patients. They were treated with 220 mg of zinc sulfate three times daily. Improvement in the time required to walk 50 feet, global assessment of disease activity, duration of morning stiffness, and joint swelling (but not tenderness) was observed. However, subsequent investigators were unable to repeat these results.

I am unaware of any scientific basis for claiming that a combination of these minerals, any combination, has any special efficacy. Of the minerals, only gold has been useful for arthritis.

Gold

For most of the 20th century, salts containing gold have existed as the leading remission-inducing drug for rheumatoid arthritis. Often but not always, they provided a reduction in active inflammation. Commonly, doses were given by weekly intramuscular injection for about 20 weeks and then gradually less frequently until a monthly regimen was achieved. Side effects consisted mainly of skin rashes, kidney impairment, and bone marrow suppression. Clinical and laboratory monitoring assured that these adverse effects were caught and the gold discontinued promptly assuring safety.

Those patients who responded well and who tolerated the gold salt injections without complication could usually be kept in partial to nearly complete remission for many months or even years with monthly injections. More recently an oral form was introduced, but it provided less effectiveness. Gold has largely been replaced by the use of methotrexate because of greater effectiveness and safety.

One study indicated that topical gold, like wearing a gold ring, was therapeutic. It was said to reduce the arthritis in the finger with the ring and in other joints near it. This has not been confirmed.

9

Foods

A young girl was admitted to an Israeli university hospital nine times over a six-year period, each time suffering from high fever, rash, and swollen, painful joints. Her diagnosis was juvenile rheumatoid arthritis. Elimination of all dairy products from her diet improved her condition dramatically, and eighteen months later she was completely free of arthritis symptoms. Juvenile rheumatoid arthritis sometimes remits spontaneously. Was this remission diet induced, or was it a spontaneous remission that was destined to occur?

A woman in London had suffered from severe rheumatoid arthritis for 25 years when her doctor discovered she had an extreme sensitivity to corn. Within a week of eliminating all corn products from her diet, she experienced remarkable improvement in her arthritis symptoms. Soon after, she went off all medication and began visiting her doctor every three months instead of weekly.

Three patients in another study experienced increased symptoms after taking capsules containing certain foods. One patient experienced increased rheumatoid arthritis symptoms after consuming milk, another experienced an inflamed joint after eating shrimp, and another patient had rheumatic aches after ingesting nitrates. However, none of the other patients in this study reacted to foods.

A food trial

Dr. R.S. Panus described the trial of a special diet in patients with rheumatoid arthritis who believed that they were allergic to a certain food or foods. This was a 10-week controlled, double blind, and randomized study of 26 patients with active rheumatoid arthritis. Eleven patients were on a specific popular diet, free of additives, preservatives, fruit, red meat, and dairy products. Fifteen were on a placebo diet. Six patients improved on the placebo diet, and five improved on the experimental diet. Improvement scores averaged 29% on placebo and 32% on the experimental diet.

While these differences are not statistically significant, two patients on the experimental diet had impressive results. They improved notably, and elected to remain on the experimental diet following the study period. They continued to improve, and subsequently, when they consumed non-experimental diet foods, they noted worsening in their arthritis.

My food study

I conducted a single blind study in which the effect of a vegan diet on rheumatoid arthritis in 12 patients was tested. All of the patients were on the vegan diet, and I was the blinded individual in this study. The team managing the study did not provide a control group simply because an adequate number of volunteers couldn't be found. Interestingly, the patients all felt better on the vegan diet, and in spite of the inconvenience it presented, several stayed on the diet for at least several months afterward. This was not a controlled study, so we need to interpret cautiously, but clinically it was impressive.

Essential fatty acids

The one food that maintains substantial scientific evidence of effectiveness is fish oil. Multiple well-designed, controlled studies support the value of omega-3 fatty acids in improving the pain, swelling, and stiffness of rheumatoid arthritis. The dose is high and the benefits are modest, but this food is also heart healthy. Remember that oil is a fat with nine calories per gram. The studies used capsules of fish oil and the dose was high enough that the patients gained weight on it. If you can enjoy fish, use it in your diet. Oily fish like salmon and mackerel are best for this. The saying now is, "A mackerel a day keeps the rheumatologist away."

Anti-inflammatory and immunosuppressive effects have been demonstrated with omega-3 and omega-6 fatty acids. Borage seed oil is a rich source of the omega-6, gamma-linoleic acid (GLA). This fatty acid was compared to a placebo of cottonseed oil in 37 patients with rheumatoid arthritis, showing a significant reduction in the number of tender joints, the severity of tenderness, and the swollen joint score. Minor intestinal discomfort was noted in a few patients with borage seed oil. Another study of 56 patients with rheumatoid arthritis compared six months of treatment with GLA to a placebo of sunflower oil. Again the GLA treated patients had significant decreases in swelling and pain. Belching and diarrhea were side effects of both GLA and sunflower oil.

Black currant seed oil contains GLA as well as the omega-3 fatty acids alpha-linoleic acid and stearidonic acid. It was associated with modest but statistically significant reduction of joint pain and swelling in a study of 34 rheumatoid arthritis patients. A placebo of soybean oil provided comparison.

Fish oil is rich in omega-3 fatty acids. It has been tested in several studies with rheumatoid arthritis. Modest but statistically significant improvements in joint pain and swelling have been documented and confirmed by several different investigators. But remember the nine calories per gram. The dose of fish oil required to produce the benefits will cause weight gain.

Enthusiasm for things natural

Enthusiasm for using natural things, especially foods, to help manage disease is impressive and as far as I can tell, universal. Daily we read about foods that will help prevent cancer or heart disease. It is only natural to want to take advantage of normal dietary items to improve our health. However, food is not medicine. A healthy diet will help maintain health, but it not a cure, despite determination to claim otherwise. More specific to our subject, foods cannot cure arthritis no matter how hard we wish they would.

One unscientific, multi-page flier offered to provide in less than five minutes, five foods that can cause you to eat away your arthritic pains like a miracle. It promises to provide the names of specific foods that give marvelous relief to arthritis and rheumatism sufferers.

As testimonial, the author offers a method for self-cure that if followed, can cure arthritis or rheumatism. But he then admits that there is no cure for arthritis or rheumatism, and asks, "Why should you suffer when you can join the many who have found freedom from pain with this natural method?". At this point anyone would be confused.

This promoter's special method is a diet that contains five special foods. First is the oil of a common nut, which he doesn't name, that will help your rheumatism or arthritis, improve your general vitality, clear up your complexion, and make your hair shine. Second is a pleasant-tasting oil that is effective in relieving symptoms of rheumatism and arthritis by helping the body absorb a certain nutrient.

Third is a common grain product that, according to recent laboratory research contains large amounts of a powerful anti-stiffness factor and is also a powerful detoxifying agent. It helps provide resistance to disease, and is especially effective in arthritis, fibrositis, neuritis, and bronchitis. Fourth is a delicious fruit that was recommended by a relative. Fifth, you have to buy his book to learn more. And that is the whole point of the brochure. He has dropped enough crumbs, he hopes, to make you follow him to the cash register. I suspect that if you did buy his book and try his formula, that you wouldn't get any relief or cure of your arthritis. He simply hopes to make enough money to make his deception worthwhile.

Food supplements

In December of 2002, the Food and Drug Administration (FDA) warned the $17 billion dietary supplement industry that it would no longer allow food supplement companies to continue to make fraudulent health claims about their products. Claims for example, that a supplement could provide a viable treatment for herpes, or has anti-viral or anti-bacterial properties, implying that they will be effective against a viral or bacterial illness would not be adequate. Pseudo science officially became insufficient. Peer-reviewed scientific study reports to support claims must now be provided before such claims may be published. As a case in point, a scientific consensus that the fiber in oatmeal helps maintain low cholesterol levels was required to be demonstrated before it could be claimed in print. Or if lacking consensus, qualified health claims must be demonstrated. A qualified health claim exists if there is a significant amount of scientific research supporting the nutrient's effect.

There was great protest when the FDA first began to warn that they were going to crack down on the supplement industry, and many petitions were circulated and signed. Now more people are recognizing the value of the FDA's oversight, especially when we read about such cases as the woman who ingested chaparral and needed a liver transplant.

Apple cider vinegar and honey

Apple cider vinegar and honey are promoted in books sold in magazines and newspapers as a treatment for arthritis and a wide range of ailments from aging, to pain, earache, indigestion, and lack of memory. Initially, I thought that this was an amusing and representative piece of folk medicine that might have been popular back in our country's pioneer days when doctors weren't available and people had to do what they could with what they had. I was obliged to change my opinion when I discovered that people today were taking it seriously. Some of the claims I have seen, listed below, fall into the too-good-to-be-true category.

Apple cider vinegar is claimed to provide relief for the following:

- chronic fatigue
- overweight and underweight
- body toxicity
- headaches
- corns, calluses, and warts
- sore throat and laryngitis
- skin problems, including symptoms of aging
- insect stings, bites, yeasts, and fungus
- dandruff, itchy scalp, dry and thinning hair, and baldness
- muscle soreness, muscle cramps
- aching joints, overall stiffness

- aging joints and connective tissues

- weak heart

- kidney and bladder problems

- gallstones

- enlarged prostate

- female troubles

- arthritis

- excessive mucus

- nose bleeds

- constipation

- abnormal blood pressure

- elevated acid crystals that cause premature aging

Too good to be true? Some foods make a difference, most don't. Some of what is promoted as therapeutic food is not based on scientific documentation but once again on wishful thinking, make-believe, or quackery.

10

Insects, Snakes, Chickens and Sharks

From ancient times, people have attempted to use all manner of animals and animal secretions to treat human diseases. In most cases, the effectiveness of these treatments has not held up to scientific scrutiny.

Centipedes

Because centipedes have many legs, they have been used for leg problems in Korean folk medicine. Insects and other arthropods have been employed in folk medicine since antiquity. Many arthropods have venom and other defensive chemicals, which are biologically active, and some have been tested and even used.

Bee sting

Bee sting or apitherapy is an old treatment for rheumatoid arthritis. Bee venom contains several proteins that have physiologic effects. Test tube experiments suggest that one of them, melitin, may slow the inflammatory response by scavenging free radicals and inhibiting the reactive oxygen species. Another theory is that the bee sting stimulates release of corticosteroids by the patient's adrenal glands. An animal model of rheumatoid arthritis known as rat adjuvant disease can be suppressed by bee venom in laboratory experiments.

Dr. Joseph Hollander, one of the great leaders of American rheumatology, reported the first controlled trial of the efficacy of bee venom in chronic arthritis and concluded that it was ineffectual. Twenty-four rheumatoid arthritis patients were treated with venom solutions injected into the skin twice each week over the most painful joints. Each patient received the equivalent of 10-30 bee stings per visit over an average of 18 sessions. Controls consisted of 9 rheumatoid arthritis patients who were injected with a milk protein mixture. Improvement occurred in 7 of 24 (29%) venom-treated patients and in 3 of 9 (33%) milk protein-treated patients. Venom was considered not effective. Improvement was lacking also in osteoarthritis and mixed types of arthritis.

Ants

Chinese ant extract preparations are a traditional Chinese medicine used mainly as a health food or drink for the treatment of rheumatism, rheumatoid arthritis, chronic hepatitis, sexual dysfunction, and anti-aging. They have been shown to be active as reactive oxygen scavengers. A partially purified extract of the South American tree ant, Psuedomyrmex, was tried in the treatment of rheumatoid arthritis. Fifteen patients received the extract and 15 received placebo. Swelling improved more than pain. Adverse effects appeared in all the venom-treated patients, including local skin reactions, fever, and chills. However, the results are difficult to interpret because anti-inflammatory drug therapy was reintroduced two weeks after initiation of ant venom injections.

Snakes

The symbol of medicine, the caduceus, is a central wand twined by two snakes, one representing evil, and the other the curative power of the viper itself. Interest in viper venoms as potential sources of anti-inflammatory substances is at once ancient and modern. It was resurrected in the 1960s by the discovery that injecting a purified protein component of venom from the cobra (naja naja) activated the complement cascade, and temporarily depleted the terminal (C3-9) components.

The complement cascade is a sort of chain reaction that occurs as a part of the immune response, and is a critical part of immune destruction of invading organisms. The cascade ends in attachment of the terminal components on the cell wall of the invading organism. When these are all attached, they break open the cell wall and the contents leak out, killing the cell. So the venomous protein blunts the complement cascade, and this blunts certain inflammatory reactions.

Data from many experimental studies indicate that in animals, cobra venom prevents or delays the onset of experimental arthritis, but it fails to improve inflammation or alter the course of established arthritis. Doses of venom large enough to cause a clinical effect also stimulate the release of corticosteroids and this causes symptomatic relief by inhibiting inflammation.

When it was applied in life, the trauma of being bitten and the associated risks of gangrene, shock, renal failure, fever, and pain associated with a cobra bite tended to discourage further complaints to the treating physician about the pain of arthritis.

Desiccated rattlesnake is used as a folk remedy for arthritis and other conditions. Two reports have been

published of serious infections in multiple patients with
Salmonella arizonae: one from Mexico City, and one from
Los Angeles. Rattlesnakes are a reservoir for this type of
Salmonella. The patients in these reports who were
infected tended to be previously immunologically
disadvantaged by AIDS, diabetes, rheumatoid arthritis,
lupus, or cancer.

Chicken collagen type II

Dr. David Trentham and his associates at Boston's
Brigham and Women's Hospital reported a placebo-
controlled double blind study with pepsin-digested type
II collagen from chickens in 60 patients with rheumatoid
arthritis. They found significant improvement in painful
and swollen joints in the patient group that received
collagen. In a subsequent study using bovine type II
collagen given in higher doses, Sieper and associates
found a slightly higher but non-significant response rate
in the treated patients, compared with placebo-treated
patients. Another study by Barnett and colleagues also
failed to show significant effectiveness.

Shark cartilage

Preparations containing shark cartilage have demonstrated potent angiogenesis and tumor cell-growth
inhibitor effects. That means that growth of tumor cells is
obstructed by blocking growth of blood vessels in the
tumor, which are necessary for the tumor survival. While
shark cartilage is useful in some experimental applications, it has no known anti-arthritic benefit.

11

PHYSICAL METHODS

Yoga

Yoga is an ancient tradition practiced for its proposed health benefits. Garfinkel and Schumacher reviewed two limited studies that reported reduction in pain in patients with osteoarthritis of the hand and carpal tunnel syndrome. The stretching and strength improvement from yoga are beneficial, and the exercises promote muscle strengthening and improved range of motion in the joints. It is in essence, is a form of physical therapy, and that in turn is part of the basic conventional therapeutic approach to all kinds of arthritis.

T'ai Chi

T'ai Chi has been called meditation in motion. It promotes relaxation, improved strength, flexibility, and control, and serves as a low impact form of exercise for the entire body that can improve range of motion, flexibility, strength, and balance.

T'ai Chi ch'uan is a combat form of martial art. Literally translated, it means "the grand ultimate fist." It takes the form of a slow moving dance-like routine with movements that are derived from the postures of animals such as the snake, crane, dragon, and tiger. These low impact routines are referred to as forms, or sets, which require the head, neck, back, and all peripheral joints to move continuously.

These routines are believed to stimulate chi, which means energy or air. Chi is said to originate from the Dan-Tien area, just below the umbilicus (navel) and flows through channels called meridians located throughout the body. Disease is believed to result from an imbalance of chi.

Acupuncture

As a component of the health care system of China for at least 2000 years, acupuncture is based on the concept that there are patterns of energy flow through the body that are essential for health. It is believed to correct imbalances in the flow of this energy, or Qi (pronounced "chee"). This method is believed to correct imbalances in the flow of energy by the puncturing of the skin with strategically placed long thin needles. The needles are placed according to 12 primary channels or meridians and eight extra-ordinary meridians. The acupuncturist selects the appropriate sites among the approximately 360 points along the meridians. In addition to the insertion of needles, the acupuncturist may apply heat, pressure, friction, suction, or electrical stimulation to these points. Many patients say that this produces a sensation of numbness, tingling, heaviness, or soreness that is called Te qi.

In traditional Chinese medicine an acupuncture practitioner seeks to identify the nature of the imbalance in order to restore balance by selecting the appropriate acupuncture points. The modern Western acupuncturist's approach to treating pain takes into account the concepts of pain mechanisms acting via nervous, endocrine, and immune mechanisms, rather than by meridians.

A combination of the use of acupuncture needles and an electrical stimulus involves placement of the needle as determined by the ancient art of acupuncture. The influence of electroacupuncture on experimental arthritis in mice was studied. Data suggested that electroacupuncture inhibited the development of arthritis in the mice, and that the benefits were produced by suppressing immune processes and the inflammatory enzyme, cyclo-oxygenase type II.

Patients with osteoarthritis of the knee participated in a study of acupuncture at the University of Maryland. Patients randomized to acupuncture improved in measures of pain and function with significantly better results than the control group, which received only standard medical management without acupuncture.

A published review of reported studies of acupuncture in osteoarthritis identified 11 studies. The reviewers noted that the results were inconsistent and contradictory. The most rigorous studies indicated that acupuncture was no better than sham treatment. Acupuncture, diazepam (Valium), and placebo plus diazepam, were compared in 44 patients with osteoarthritis of the neck. The results indicated that acupuncture was significantly more effective than placebo plus diazepam, but not better than sham acupuncture or diazepam alone.

There have been a few studies on acupuncture for fibromyalgia, and most of them have been small and poorly controlled. One exception is a study by Deluze and colleagues, which was a randomized, controlled study in 70 fibromyalgia patients. The patients received six treatments of either electroacupuncture that elicited Te chi, or sham acupuncture (superficial needling without Te chi). Outcomes showed statistically significant improvement in the real acupuncture group versus the sham acupuncture group. Both animal and human studies have documented that endorphins are increased in the cerebral-spinal fluid after acupuncture. This would suggest that it is effective for pain control and especially for the chronic pain of fibromyalgia.

There have been limited studies on acupuncture in the treatment of rheumatoid arthritis. One of these was a randomized controlled trial, but it employed only 10 patients. This study required participation by patients who had bilateral involvement of the knees. One knee was treated with acupuncture and compared to the opposite knee which was treated with sham acupuncture. Pain relief lasted for one to three months in the treated knee, but only ten hours or less in the sham treated knee.

When patients ask me about acupuncture, I advise them that it is okay to try it, but only if they find an acupuncturist who uses sterile needles. Years ago we had a few cases of hepatitis caused by unsterilized needles, and today AIDS is another concern. Also, I request that my patients report results of the acupuncture to me. Many reported that it didn't help. Several said they felt better initially, but the effect didn't last beyond a few weeks. One or two reported that the acupuncturist advised them that acupuncture was not effective for arthritis. Patients with fibromyalgia tend to be more responsive to acupuncture.

Adverse effects can occur. In one case, an infected joint (septic arthritis of the sacroiliac joint) developed after acupuncture was administered without first cleansing the skin with alcohol. In another instance, a 74-year-old man experienced a punctured lung, causing escape of air inside the chest wall and a collapse of the lung (pneumothorax). The needle had been inserted around the base of the neck, and obviously, the technique was imprecise or worse in that case. A physician trained in acupuncture should have the knowledge that would preclude that kind of complication. Yet, at the base of the neck the proximity of the lung is an issue of risk.

Chiropractic

Manipulative relief of back or neck pain can be provided by skillful chiropractic technique. However, chiropractors do not have a full medical education, and they may not know the implications of arthritis for their manipulative efforts. This can be hazardous.

Manipulation of the neck is especially dangerous. Rheumatoid arthritis tends to involve the neck, and when it does, it is especially apt to weaken the upper neck at the joints between the first and second vertebrae. This creates a tendency for those vertebrae to slip from their proper position, making them vulnerable to sliding forward and backward. And when they do, they can compress the spinal cord. One of my patients with rheumatoid arthritis went to the chiropractor for her neck pain, received her chiropractic adjustment, and became paralyzed in all four extremities for the rest of her life.

Low back involvement with rheumatoid arthritis does occur. It is less common and less dangerous than neck involvement, but that does not mean it is entirely safe in terms of chiropractic treatments. Ankylosing spondylitis is a variant of rheumatoid arthritis that can involve the low back or the whole spine including the neck. It causes the spine to become rigid and encourages a tendency for unusual spinal fractures from excessive stresses. Any application of manipulative technique to the spine in people with rheumatoid arthritis or its variants can be risky. Therefore, the question to have answered before you see a chiropractor is: "Does my chiropractor have the training to know if I have arthritis in my back, as well as what kind it is?"

Degenerative disk disease a type of osteoarthritis, and it is a very common type of back problem. Muscle and ligament strains are even more common. In these cases the risks are less serious, and manipulation may offer some relief. Osteopathic physicians are medically educated and licensed to practice medicine. They should have the knowledge to make a correct diagnosis of arthritis, and some may also practice spinal manipulation. Consult one of these physicians if you want to pursue manipulative technique.

12

Spiritual Methods

By spiritual methods, I mean methods that involve a discipline of spirit. Relaxation, contemplation, even prayer. The mind has a powerful influence on the body.

Relaxation

For pain relief, relaxation techniques are effective. Lie down in a comfortable, quiet place with the lights low. Start with your toes. Focus on them and let them relax. Next, relax your feet. Concentrate. Work gradually from your ankles to your legs, then your knees, thighs, hips, and so on, up to your chest. Then to your hands, arms, neck and head. Most of us are asleep before we get that far. The benefits of a gentle stroking massage, cuddling, and loving also are part of the therapeutic relaxation concept, as is the appropriate use of alcohol, and aromatherapy.

Aromatherapy

Essential oils have been used for their fragrance and restorative effects on body and mind since pre-biblical times. Fragrant oils are blended to produce calmness, emotional balance, and stress relief. However, claims that they correct hormonal balance are fallacious thinking. These oils are used in a bath, or in massage oil, or dispersed into the room via an aroma diffuser or passive air freshener. Some of the benefits claimed include antibacterial effects from clary sage and eucalyptus, and an anti-inflammatory effect from frankincense, lemon, and peppermint.

One study was conducted in England with eight women and one man, all with rheumatoid arthritis. Before and after massage they were asked to complete visual analogue scales of pain, sleep, and well-being. Pain was not reduced, nor sleep improved, but following massage with lavender oil, the perception of well-being was enhanced.

Flotation Therapy

Balneotherapy or spa therapy is also called flotation therapy. Spas became popular for treating arthritis during Roman times for the likes of Julius Caesar among others. Such spas remain popular today in parts of Europe and Israel. The Dead Sea, the saltiest body of water on Earth, is so densely saline that people float in the water as therapy. And mud baths are especially popular in Calistoga, California.

Different spas have been recommended for a variety of conditions, depending on whether the water has a sulphurous, bicarbonate, or sodium chloride quality. All have been recommended for rheumatic conditions. Since most patients feel better when they are away from home and enjoying a restful and interesting vacation, one of the benefits of spas is that they are part of physical and psychological rest and recreation.

An uncontrolled study was reported by doctors Hill, Eckett, Paterson and Harkness. Fourteen people who had osteoarthritis of weight bearing joints entered the study, but four dropped out. Each received a series of six treatment sessions at approximately one-week intervals. Treatments took place at a center that had an established floatation pool in a well heated room with subdued lighting and music. The response was measured by results of three different medical status questionnaires. According to one of the questionnaires, all 10 individuals improved, but the same result was not found by using the other two questionnaires.

Therapeutic Touch

The laying-on-of-hands (not in the religious sense, although it is related) through the reassuring touch of a doctor or therapist, and/or the comforting touch of a parent or spouse is an integral part of medical care.

Beyond those forms of touch is Therapeutic Touch, which involves the active employment of the practitioner's perceptions as they move their hands an inch or two above a patient's body. A study reported in the *Journal of Family Practice* in 1998 involved 25 patients with osteoarthritis of the knee. Patients continued to receive their usual medications and care during this trial of Therapeutic Touch. The Therapeutic Touch treatment group received a treatment once a week for six weeks, while the control group received a mock treatment while the therapist focused on a cognitive task rather than on the patient. The treatment group experienced better improvement in pain and function compared to controls. No confirming studies have been reported.

Prayer

In a study reported in the December 2001 *Mayo Clinic Proceedings*, Doctors Mueller, Plevak and Rummans observed that when people consult physicians to learn the nature of their illness and its treatment, often the subtext of their enquiry is, "Why is this happening to me?" Too often the answer is not to be found in medical science, but evokes a need for spiritual or religious support. Long have religion and medicine been entwined. For many centuries building hospitals and training physicians and nurses have been an outreach of religious groups. In the study noted above, these authors reviewed published studies that examined the association between religious involvement and spirituality, physical and mental health, and health-related quality of life. They concluded that most patients have a spiritual life, regard their spiritual health and physical health equally important, and often have greater spiritual needs during illness. The authors found many studies that show a direct relationship between religious involvement, spirituality, and positive health outcomes, including a relationship to mortality, quality of living, and coping with illness.

In the same issue of the *Mayo Clinic Proceedings*, Dr. Aviles et al reported a study in which intercessory prayer was tested in a double blind manner. Patients who were admitted to a coronary care unit were randomly assigned either to a group being prayed for or a control group, not prayed for. Neither physicians nor patients knew who was being prayed for, nor did the intercessors know the patients they were praying for. Intercessory prayer by one or more persons on behalf of the patient was undertaken at least once a week for 26 weeks by 5 intercessors per patient. The results showed no significant effect of intercessory prayer on medical outcomes after hospitalization in a coronary care unit. Perhaps this has something to do with the need for the patient to be directly involved in the prayerful effort.

A 58-year-old woman with a 30 year history of rheumatoid arthritis was described by Dale A. Matthews, M.D. The woman was an Registered Nurse who had been disabled by her arthritis because of multiple severe deformities. She was unable to fully dress or bathe herself, and had much difficulty climbing a flight of stairs. She had substantial pain and was on treatment with state-of-the-art medications that included azathioprine and prednisone. She participated in a three-day intercessory prayer ministry retreat. This included six hours of educational sessions regarding the nature of healing and six hours on in-person hands-on intercessory prayer in which volunteer prayer ministers placed their hands on her affected joints and prayed aloud on her behalf for healing.

Immediately after the intervention, her self-reported levels of pain and fatigue dropped 35%, and her global sense of well-being and functional level doubled. One year after the intervention, her number of tender joints had dropped from a pre-intervention level of eight to a post-intervention level of none. The number of swollen joints dropped from three to none. Fatigue decreased and grip strength, functional ability, and sense of well-being improved. Pain was diminished and medication doses had decreased.

Dr. Matthews and associates also reported a study of the effects on rheumatoid arthritis of intercessory prayer for healing used in conjunction with standard medical treatment. Patients with long-standing, moderately severe rheumatoid arthritis were shown to have significant short- and long-term physical benefits from in-person intercessory prayer ministry. Significant overall improvement in the major outcome variables (patient-related pain, fatigue, functional status, joint tenderness, swelling and grip strength) over a twelve month period following a three day, in-person laying on of hands healing and educational intervention. Joint swelling and tenderness decreased by 68% and 66% respectively. Patient rated pain decreased by 31%.

The improvement was attributed to the addition of the complementary effects of group education, support, and counseling to the patient's medical treatment. These enhance coping, quality of life, feelings of self-worth, adjustment, happiness, usefulness, purpose in life and general well-being. The authors attributed these effects to the elicitation of the relaxation response, which in turn can trigger a reduction in stress, enhancement of immune functioning and provision of hope. Depression and anxiety are overcome. Social networks are augmented and unhealthy behaviors are reduced. Rituals and sacraments have an atmosphere of love and beauty. Feelings central to prayer include love, empathy, compassion, and a sense of connectedness.

13

The Newest Probably Effective Complementary Alternatives

Glucosamine and Chondroitin

Glucosamine sulfate, often combined with chondroitin sulfate, was initially marketed with the gloss and fanfare of an unproven remedy. Careful, double-blind, placebo-controlled studies held both before and after it was marketed in the United States remain inconsistent, but ultimately many investigators have documented evidence that patients with osteoarthritis experience significant relief by taking it. Also, current studies appear to support promoters' claims that these agents help build and repair cartilage damaged by the disease. Initially, investigators in Europe documented their studies, and since then reports have been filed in the United States, Canada, and around the world. The studies have been appropriate, well designed, and supportive.

Glucosamine for osteoarthritis was reviewed in the September 26, 1997, edition of *The Medical Letter* (a highly respected review of current clinical pharmacology) and concluded that it appeared to be safe. Some patients, the review stated, had complained of nausea or gastrointestinal discomfort, but it was no more or less frequent with glucosamine than with the placebo. The undocumented purity of the available products was a concern. Some of the studies had reported beneficial effects, but reviewers were not convinced of its effectiveness, because they felt the eight-week studies were too brief.

Since 1997, numerous studies and reviews have been published in medical literature. During the two years between 1999 and 2002, 140 articles were published in English, including reviews, commentaries, and at least 40 randomized clinical trials of glucosamine. Many other studies did not go to print, including the study I conducted.

In my practice, we studied the effect of 500mg of glucosamine three times daily for six weeks. We measured the effect of this dosage in 40 patients with osteoarthritis of the knee, and compared it to 40 patients who received a placebo instead. Pain was the main sign of disease activity. Most of the patients got better, and since the placebo patients improved as much as the glucosamine patients, we were able to see no difference.

My study coincided with major media hype about the benefits of glucosamine. At the same time, there were many articles and headlines about it in newspapers and national magazines, and TV news programs discussed it repeatedly. I believe that this attention produced a mass placebo effect that confounded the study. Therefore, I felt our results were misleading and decided not to publish them.

One of the better clinical trials was published in Clinical Therapeutics in 1980. This study, reported by italian doctors Drovanti, Bignamini, and Rovati, measured joint pain, tenderness, swelling, and restriction of motion in 80 patients for 30 days. There were 40 patients in the glucosamine group, and 40 in the placebo group. Compared to the results on placebo, glucosamine was associated with statistically greater improvement in pain, tenderness, swelling, and both active and passive knee movement. When combined, the scores recorded for each of these measures of disease showed a 72% reduction of symptoms in the glucosamine group and 36% on placebo.

A glucosamine-osteoarthritis study

Nine orthopedic and rheumatology clinics participated in a study of patients who had osteoarthritis with pain, but without swelling or inflammation. These patients were divided into two groups of 120 and 121, both groups taking two sugar-coated tablets three times a day. The group of 120 received glucosamine sulfate, and the group of 121 received the placebo. The Lequesne index was used to compare results, and the Lequesne score averaged 10.6 for both glucosamine treated patients and for those who received the placebo. Nonetheless, this showed a statistically insignificant decrease in the Lequesne score of 3.2 points for the glucosamine group and 2.2 points for the placebo group.

Overall, a clinical response suggesting improvement was recorded in 58% of patients on glucosamine, and 38% of those on placebo. None of the differences between glucosamine and placebo reached statistical significance, except for the overall clinical response difference of 58% compared to 38%. This provides little or no meaningful support for the effectiveness of glucosamine because the individual indicators of effectiveness failed to differentiate glucosamine from placebo.

Glucosamine and its role in joint health

Glucosamine is one of the principal components of several important ingredients of cartilage and of the synovial fluid that bathes and lubricates the joint. Glucosamine is a major building block of the glycosaminoglycans and hyaluronic acid, which hold the cartilage together, give it sponginess and an ability to hold water, and lubricate the two cartilage surfaces as they rub against each other. Chondroitin sulfate is similar to glucosamine and has the same general properties.

Glucosamine is believed to stimulate biosynthesis of the proteoglycan molecules that serve as a structural component in cartilage. These are extremely long, winding molecules that wind around pillars made of collagen and act as a glue, holding things in place. These molecules also have a high negative charge, allowing them to hold water that squeezes out under muscle pressure or weight bearing. When the weight or pressure is released from the joint, the water is absorbed back into the cartilage like a sponge. While the water is in the joint, it mixes with the joint fluid. Thus it is exchanged for fresh fluid that contains nutrients. When the water is sucked back into the cartilage, it carries oxygen and nutrients to the cartilage cells. Since there are no blood vessels in cartilage, this is how the cartilage gets its nourishment.

When pressure squeezes water out of the cartilage, the water also forms a lining on the surface of the cartilages between the ends of two bones, which provides a slippery or lubricated surface. Glucosamine is a component of hyaluronate in the joint fluid that increases joint slipperiness. Also, in osteoarthritis, whether it is primary or secondary to rheumatoid arthritis, proteoglycans are broken down and depleted. Continuing research supports the impression that glucosamine is taken up in the cartilage and plays a role in maintaining the proteoglycans. Glucosamine may have other protective effects, like blocking the damaging effects of reactive oxygen and nitrogen radicals and lysosomal enzymes produced during inflammation.

But does it work?

Beyond symptomatic relief, and despite efforts to document it, does any evidence demonstrate that glucosamine and chondroitin sulfate actually inhibit the structural damage inherent in the progression of osteoarthritis? Does the pill you swallow really end up in the cartilage? The answer is yes. Radio labeled glucosamine studies reveal that ultimately it does end up in the joint cartilage. Laboratory evidence points as well to the employment of glucosamine in maintaining cartilage viability.

Two longer term studies have recently been reported. They both support the clinical benefits of glucosamine. The first of these appeared in *The Lancet* in January 2001. Authored by a team of 10 physicians lead by Jean Yves Reginster, M.D., this study involved 212 patients with osteoarthritis of the knee. Divided into two groups of 106 patients each, they received either 1500 mg of oral glucosamine or placebo once daily for three years. All of the placebo patients had progressive loss of cartilage over the three years of the study. There was no significant cartilage loss in the 106 patients who received glucosamine. Symptoms worsened slightly over the three years in the placebo group, but improvement was observed after receiving glucosamine.

The second recent long term study appeared in the *Archives of Internal Medicine* on October 14, 2002. Karel Pavelka, M.D., Ph.D. and a team of six physicians reported another three year study that compared glucosamine 1500 mg a day and placebo. There were 101 patients in each group. There was a progressive loss of cartilage space in the knees of those on placebo but not for those on glucosamine. Symptoms improved even with placebo but they improved more with glucosamine.

Shopping for glucosamine

When shopping for glucosamine, you'll find a bewildering array of products—tablets, capsules, creams, and liquids—with fanciful names that seem to promise huge benefits. The prices range from around $12 for 90 capsules of glucosamine 500 mg. to $60 for 90 capsules of combinations containing glucosamine-chondroitin sulfate, MSM, and SAM-e. Which should you choose?

Save your money. I'll tell you why.

Methylsulfonylmethane (MSM)

Promotional material for MSM says the initials stand for methylsulfonylmethane. This, they claim, is a natural sulfur compound found in all living things. That much is true. It's one of the most prominent compounds in our bodies, ranking right behind water and salt. But, if that's so, how can we be deficient in it?

The list of effects and claims for MSM is long, diverse, and imprecise:

- It's safe because the sulfur in MSM is sulfonyl, which is different from bad sulfurs like sulfas, sulfates, sulfites, and sulfides.

- It isn't a drug or a medicine, but MSM improves such health problems as allergies, asthma, emphysema, lung dysfunction, arthritis, headaches, skin problems, stomach and digestive tract problems, circulation, cell osmosis, and absorption.

- MSM acts as an analgesic and anti-inflammatory.

- It inhibits muscle spasm and increases blood flow.

- It's found in common foods such as raw milk, meat, fish, fruits, grains, and vegetables.

- But it's lacking in our diet, because it's processed out.

- It's highly active, which is why it has so many benefits.

- It has no side effects.

- It's "safer than water."

That many effects, and that lack of precision, raises the specter of many side effects, and raises the equally problematic question: Does it have any effects? Interestingly, *there isn't one published scientific study that demonstrates any validity to the claims made for MSM. None.*

SAM-e

The nutriceutical called SAM-e (S-adenosyl-L-methionine), pronounced "Sammy," is utilized in three important metabolic pathways, all of which are important in normal cell function and survival. Interference of any of these pathways or normal reactions can affect cell processes and the body's healthy survival. Given the importance of these roles, it is easy to understand why this compound has been the focus of substantial investigation.

A search for this nutriceutical on the Web brought almost 60,000 hits. Most claims are for its use for depression, and far fewer for joint pain. Studies have focused largely on its use as an antidepressant, and for treating alcohol induced liver disease. The results for arthritis have been disappointing. In one arthritis study at the University of Indiana, patients with osteoarthritis seemed to benefit initially, but by the end of the study, any benefit had evaporated. Placebo and SAM-e each produced similar results.

In another placebo-controlled study, there were two groups at different sites. One group, with less severe osteoarthritis had less pain than the placebo treated controls at the end of 28 days of treatment with SAM-e.

The patients in the second site had more severe disease and they fared no better than their placebo control partners.

Capsaicin

Capsaicin, made from hot chili peppers, is popular and reasonably effective in relieving pain in joints, ligaments, muscles, and tendons. It is applied topically as a cream, lotion, or deodorant-like stick and is absorbed rapidly. It reduces pain sensation and transmission to the brain, and it inhibits the inflammatory process. It causes the C-fiber pain sensory neurons to become unexcitable and it inactivates the release of neuropeptides from peripheral nerve endings. While it relives pain, it can cause a temporary hot or burning sensation. The best product comes in an applicator bottle, so you needn't get it on your hands in applying it. It is especially irritating to eyes, and to mucous membranes like the mouth and the genitalia if you touch these areas after getting it on your hand. And it lasts on your hand for hours. It is applied lightly over the area to be treated three or four times a day for at least three weeks.

Caveat emptor

Testimonials for products like those above are unreliable, because often as not, or maybe more often than not, they are written by some ad agency and not by a customer at all. Also, in the case of products sold through pyramid companies, it's too easy to be led to believe in a product, buy it, and try it, and waste money on it, because a friend urges us to. Be careful why you buy and try. You may do no more than waste money, or worse, consume something that does you some real harm. Before you buy and try something, seek written, verifiable, scientific proof of the products value. After all, don't you check with *Consumer Reports* or a knowledgeable expert before you buy a toaster or a TV? When an uncredentialed salesperson at the local store advises you, are you getting valid advice? When it is about your health, ask someone reliable, with the right background, who is not dependant on the sale for his or her income. Ask your rheumatologist.

Placebo Effect

Sometimes quack cures seem to work. How can that be? Arthritis, like many diseases can wax and wane spontaneously. So, when we take a remedy and feel better, we become convinced that the remedy is the cure. This is why we hold large studies with many patients and compare the effects of the new or tested remedy to a known non-effective substance called a placebo. Placebo pills or capsules are made to look just like the remedy being tested, and taste, odor, and appearance are disguised. Neither the doctor doing the test, nor the patients participating in the study can know who gets the active remedy and who receives the placebo. Then, when the study is completed, the code is broken and the results of remedy are compared to the results of placebo. If results reveal a difference in favor of the remedy, it must be repeated elsewhere, by different doctors and on different patients, to confirm that the first results were not accidentally skewed.

In any double-blind, controlled trial, about a third of the patients who receive the placebo, even under double blind conditions, respond well at least temporarily. This is the "placebo effect." It may represent coincidental spontaneous waning of the disease or it may be a psychological response where the subconscious mind convinces the conscious mind that the product is performing as desired. One tongue in cheek admonition: avoid taking too many placebos; you may become permanently duped. The mind is powerful, and in a situation where we're seeking arthritis relief, both patient and investigator want the benefit to happen, and the mind makes it so, at least temporarily. Real relief would be longer lasting.

What's wrong with having a placebo effect? The placebo effect is nice, if it gives you temporary relief from a temporary problem. If the problem is long-lasting, any relief is better than none. But the fact that it doesn't last is disappointing and discouraging when you thought you might finally have found the relief you had sought. But more than disappointment, it's possible that you might be discouraged from seeking real, substantive relief. While arthritis has been an affliction of the human race for thousands of years, and substantive relief is only recent, we are making huge scientific progress in finding relief and steps are being made toward cures.

Beyond the placebo effect is the fraudulent practice of using counterfeit or unsubstantiated ideas or claims to promote a product known to be worthless. Whether fraud is at work in the claims discussed here is a matter of conjecture. My doubts are based in judgment developed in years of study and experience. The validity of my doubts and the integrity of the claims and the claimants described are subject to validation by objective scientific investigation. When objective validation is presented, we should all review it with an open mind, but until it is offered, be wary.

The problem with unproved remedies is that they ensnare a substantial number of people, and huge amounts of money. Right now, when we're struggling to reduce the cost of legitimate medicine, it's estimated that we're spending $10 billion a year on unproved remedies in the United States alone. This emphasizes the interest in finding natural products that can enhance our health. It is a mistake to think that there are hidden cures, but I think few people are looking for just that. I think we feel that if we can do something simple, inexpensive, and safe, in addition to obtaining good medical care that will enhance our health, we want to do that.

To put it into perspective, I have described some interesting unproved remedies. My intent is to provide you with a point of reference to help you understand where alternative therapies fit. I have searched the scientific literature electronically by using the Medlars system that you can access through National Library of Medicine program at www.pubmed.nl. I have presented the best evidence I could find in support of the alternative therapies I discuss. The tremendous interest in self-help therapies is important and understandable. Self-reliance is, after all, part of our American heritage. And, of course, I will explore the benefits of the ultimate in alternative therapy, meaning of course, sex and alcohol.

The Ultimate Alternatives

This you can believe:

- Complementary and alternative treatments are to be used in addition to medical treatment, not instead of it.

- A single well-controlled study is not reliable until confirmed by more well-controlled studies.

- Anecdotal reports are not reliable.

- Successful treatments earn billions. No one keeps them secret.

- Even water has side effects. Trying unproved remedies risks potential side effects.

- Keep an open mind, but don't be fooled by false hopes.

The ultimate alternatives just might be sex and alcohol!

14

FDA Approved Medicines For Arthritis

The Food and Drug Administration (FDA) is the American regulatory agency charged with ensuring that medicines are effective and safe—that patients are not exposed to unknown side effects. A side effect is something that occurs but was not planned or sought. Sometimes a side effect can be beneficial; usually it is not. Almost anything we do carries such a potential.

Side Effects and Safety

Driving to and from your doctor's office carries more risk than taking the prescription the doctor writes. To lower the risk in both instances, pay attention to the rules and instructions. In the case of medical treatment, notify the doctor if something unexpected happens, and keep your follow-up appointments so your doctor can monitor your response to treatment. Don't fear side effects to medication any more than you fear side effects to driving a car, but respect both.

When testing new medicines, before and after they are marketed, doctors in the clinic, in the pharmaceutical company, and at the FDA, remain focused on identifying any unforeseen side effects. Dangerous side effects are cause for denying approval of a new drug application. No legitimate medication can be marketed without documented safety. While it's possible for unanticipated side effects to appear after use is widespread, most are known well before you fill your prescription. Once you do, it pays to be attentive because side effects generally make their presence known boldly. Thus, in terms of safety, treat medicines with the same care and respect that you give to crossing the street or driving a car.

Hyaluronate

Hyaluronic acid derivatives afford help for osteoarthritis. Hyaluronate sodium (Hyalgan^R, or Supartz^R) is a viscous solution of one of the main components of joint fluid, and Hylan^R G-F 20 (Synvisc^R) is even thicker. Injected into the joint, these medicines offer excellent relief from pain and swelling in early to moderate osteoarthritis. When they are effective, the benefit tends to last for many months, the injections may be repeated as needed, and they can keep you out of the operating room. Your rheumatologist or orthopedist can determine if these medicines are appropriate for you and, if so, to do the injections they require.

NSAIDs and Cox-II Blockers

For most rheumatologic diseases, including osteoarthritis and rheumatoid arthritis, anti-inflammatory drugs like ibuprofen (Motrin^R) or naproxen (Naprosyn^R, Aleve^R) are valuable. More recently, safer Cox II anti-inflammatory medicines like celecoxib (Celebrex^R), rofecoxib (Vioxx^R) and valdicoxib (Bextra^R) have been introduced. The list of these anti-inflammatory medicines is long. They work by blocking an enzyme involved in joint inflammation and by relieving pain.

Ibuprofen and naproxen are available in over-the-counter strengths without a prescription. They are very helpful and generally safe, except that some people get excessive stomach or bowel irritation from them that can cause serious bleeding. The Cox II inhibitors are less irritating to the stomach and intestine, but even they are occasionally associated with gastrointestinal bleeding.

When you need to use either of these, be alert to excessive heartburn or diarrhea, and if you notice a black stool, report it to your doctor immediately. Black means black, not just dark. It is a sign of digested blood and of iron in the stool. If you are taking iron pills, the black color should already be there before you take these medicines, confusing the issue.

Occasionally these medicines can cause water retention and swelling, and possibly a small rise in blood pressure. Significant blood pressure rise is rare. Adverse effects on the kidneys or liver are rare. If you require these anti-inflammatory drugs on a frequent or ongoing basis, these considerations are good reason to have your physician follow your progress.

There were clues that the Cox II inhibitors might also reduce the risk of recurrence of colon polyps. The manufacturer (Merck) began a study to evaluate this and in the process they observed a small but serious increased risk of heart attacks in patients taking rofecoxib (Vioxx[R]). They promptly reported this finding and voluntarily removed rofecoxib from the market. This finding confirmed suspicions raised in several earlier studies. Overall, the data from these studies indicate that the relative risk of cardiovascular complications appears to be 1.0, meaning no increased risk for patients taking celecoxib, 1.29 for rofecoxib in a dose of 25mg daily, 3.15 with rofecoxib in a dose of 50 mg daily and 1.16 with the older non-steroidal anti-inflammatory drugs. More investigation is ongoing.

Cortisone and Remission-Inducing Drugs

In the 1950s, the Mayo Clinic's Nobel Prize winner Philip Hench, M.D., discovered that cortisone (prednisone) can provide dramatic relief from the severe inflammation, pain, and swelling of rheumatoid arthritis. At about the same time, a series of remission-inducing drugs were introduced that are able to decrease the severity of rheumatoid arthritis. Their effectiveness varies, and their benefits last for variable periods. These remission-inducing drugs include gold salts, antimalarial drugs, penicillamine, sulfasalazine, azathioprine, methotrexate, and cyclosporine. Added to the list most recently is leflunomide (Arava), which has an impressive ability to induce remissions of rheumatoid arthritis.

Cortisone is not used, but its variations, like prednisone, are. It is a life-saver in the sense that it saves lives and it saves quality of life for those with severe arthritis. It is capable of dramatic effects, both therapeutic and adverse. The risks include water and salt retention, swelling, obesity, hypertension, and osteoporosis. Despite these adverse effects it is often necessary, but generally it is used in the lowest dose that will do the job and for the shortest time possible. Unfortunately, for some patients the shortest time is a very long time. Fortunately, the remission inducing drugs can significantly reduce the need for prednisone.

Dramatic new biological remission inducing drugs

Most recently, precise and effective designer drugs have appeared that are biological agents for rheumatoid arthritis. Our understanding of the processes involved in the immune response system has grown, and the mechanisms of inflammation and tissue damage are understood better. Thus, we can pinpoint specific steps in the process and interrupt them precisely. This permits greater accuracy in effectiveness and marked reduction of side effects. These new medicines include the TNF (tumor necrosis factor) blockers: infliximab (Remicade[R]), etanercept (Enbrel[R]), adalimumab (Humira[R]), and the interleukin-1 blocker, IL-1 RA (Anakinra[R]). They are true remission-inducing drugs, capable of stopping or profoundly interrupting the progressive damage to the joints that is the hallmark of rheumatoid arthritis. This is the huge breakthrough we have been waiting for, and there are more new therapies of this kind in the pipeline.

My perspective

The new biological disease modifying antirheumatic drugs can halt the progression of damage in the joints. This means that they prevent crippling. That is nothing short of thrilling. And more are on the way. Not just new versions of the same things, but whole new approaches that either block cytokine messenger proteins that promote damage, or mimic other cytokines that are protective.

With the ability to halt the progress of rheumatoid arthritis, and to limit the symptoms and perhaps the progress of osteoarthritis, it is more important now than ever that people with arthritis seek the help of a qualified specialist in rheumatology. The use of complementary and alternative therapies will certainly continue. Stick to those with merit and avoid the snake oils. And remember the "ultimate" alternatives...

15

The Importance of Sex

The importance of sex was described well and entertainingly by Mark Twain in his book, *Letters from the Earth: Uncensored Writings by Mark Twain,* Edited by Bernard DeVoto (1991). Twain writes as Satan, the celestial day is equivalent to 1000 years of our time, and Satan is a close companion of Archangels Michael and Gabriel.

Apparently, Satan has been making admiring asides (often biting and always funny), to his friends the other Archangels about certain of the Creator's sparkling industries. Twain's remarks are satirical, his favored literary form. When Satan's comments were overheard by some ordinary angels and reported to Headquarters, he was given a celestial day's banishment, something that had happened before. Formerly, he'd been deported into space for his time-outs since there was nowhere else to send him, and he'd flapped about tediously in the arctic chill of eternal night. This time he decided to push on to find Earth and see how the human-race experiment was coming along. After a time, he writes about it to Saints Michael and Gabriel.

Twain's narrative is acerbic, accurate, and droll. I wanted to quote several passages for you on these pages, but could not get permission, so I can only urge you to read the book, which was re-released in 1991. In *Letters From Earth*, Twain remarks about what an odd place Earth is, and what an even odder creation is man, who has the temerity to think himself as the "noblest work of God." And he imagines that heaven is a place in which sexual intercourse, the most heavenly of delights, does not exist. Twain is aghast. "Man," says Satan, "is a marvel," and wonders who invented this oddity?

Mark Twain is a marvel himself, in my opinion. No one has described human nature more incisively or with more humor, spiced with well aimed mockery. Sex is a powerful biologic force that is bound not only to physical urge, but to equally important psychological needs for consortium. The intimate relationship between lovers is motivating, rewarding, and fulfilling. It is the natural source of life's greatest happiness.

Sex is motivating

Through much of our young lives, the physical pleasure of sex permeates our thoughts. Consider how much time people think about sex, or girl- or guy-watching? Sex in advertising is directed at both men and women. Think of Victoria's Secret, Calvin Klein, or any magazine. Sex influences what we wear and how we wear it. It pervades our entertainment, movies, television, music, all of life.

Songs go a step deeper, revealing the underlying truth that there is more to sex than intercourse, showing that the equally important emotional part that relates to affection is the *heart* of the intimate relationship.

Yes, sex is sexual, intimately sexual, but it is more. It is deeper than copulation, and that is how it motivates us to behave in attractive ways in order to be seen both as physically attractive, and warm and caring. This motivating element conveys the intimacy of sex and the psychological element of relationship.

Sex is rewarding

The physical rewards are obvious, but the rewards that make the relationship soar in importance are the harvest of the intimate relationship. This harvest produced by the intimate relationship is support, counsel, sharing, understanding, laughter, empathy, companionship to share in good times and bad. When the intimate relationship leads to establishing a family, all of the advantages, motivational forces, and rewards associated with the intimate relationship are magnified hundreds of times.

The intimate relationship is fulfilling. It allows one to grow beyond oneself, to live and breathe for each other. By that, I don't mean to lose one's self in the other, but to be 50% of the relationship, but together to be 200% when sharing the moments of beauty, and shouldering together the inevitable responsibilities in raising a family. Thus is growth expanded and fulfillment magnified.

We need our intimate relationships

Married couples live longer, and in better health. For example, a man lived to be 100 years. When his friends asked him how he explained his longevity, he said that when he and his wife were first married they made an agreement that whenever they had an argument, one of them would leave the house. "I attribute my long life," he said, "to having lived an outdoor life."

Rheumatic diseases and sex

In the textbook *Rheumatic Diseases: Diagnosis and Management*, edited by Warren A. Katz, M.D., he wrote a chapter entitled "Sexuality and Arthritis." There he notes that, because people are reluctant to talk about sex, there have been few formal investigations of the sexual problems of people with arthritis, and he reviewed some that had been published.

In one study, over half of the 45 subjects with disabilities, including arthritis, indicated that their handicap caused a change in the frequency of sexual activity. To a lesser extent, mutual satisfaction and interest also declined.

He quoted a study by Currey, who showed that 25 percent of 121 patients with osteoarthritis of the hip experienced sexual difficulties, and that arthritis produced a definite unhappiness or tension in their marriages. The frequency of marital discord was proportional to the degree of sexual difficulty.

Dr. Katz wrote further that the positive effects of sex on arthritis also need to be considered. In a loving sexual relationship, an essential part is that someone cares. This caring allows for deeper and freer communication. It allows freedom to vent frustrations and offer support for concerns as well as the opportunity to share happiness and success.

On occasion, patients have told to me that they have less pain after sex. In conference at a recent national meeting of the American College of Rheumatology, a Registered Nurse participant with rheumatoid arthritis testified that she feels much better and has less pain for a day after having sex. The effect of sex on arthritis is covered in the next chapter, but for now, let's look at the effect of arthritis on sex and sexuality.

It is safe to presume that arthritis can produce physical barriers to any physical activity, including sexual intercourse? Yes and no. We must not rule out or forget compensation, creativity, compassion, and consideration.

Let us apply an old New England rule of thumb: With arthritis, "you can do anything that doesn't make it worse afterward." It is good to explore. Sometimes the libido suffers from the pain and fatigue of arthritis, as well as offering a loss of self-image from the physical manifestations of arthritis. More than it should, according to the evidence I have seen, but then self-image is not always built on accurate data.

But self-image is a perception that is magnified by the depression that comes from the combined emotional and physical impediments of the disease. And a loving, compassionate sexual relationship can go a long way to improve these emotional effects of arthritis. Patients need healthy relationships to be all they are capable of being. Sexual interplay, combined with hugging, kissing, stroking, talking, and massage are adjuncts and alternatives that are as meaningful and satisfying as intercourse. A healthy sexual relationship supports a fulfilling life, and makes it possible to enjoy all the aspects of one's humanity.

Arthritis patients and their spouses should communicate with their physician about the frustrations and handicaps they experience. Too often people are reluctant to talk to the doctor about sexual experiences, and doctors, too, tend to be wary about intruding on the patients' privacy. That door needs to be opened.

My perspective

Sexuality is a core, meaningful, and essential part of our lives. Too often it is neglected in settings of medical care. Reticence about discussing sexual matters is an issue for both patient and physician. Since it is meaningful, and important, and universal, we need to drop our social squeamishness and face it honestly.

16

What Arthritis Does to Sex

A number of studies have documented how rheumatoid arthritis intrudes on sexual relationships. "The sexual quality of life in rheumatoid arthritis," a study by Ferguson and Figley, found that 54% of women and 56% of men with arthritis had sexual problems due to pain or weakness, problems with a partner, and/or fatigue.

Yoshino and Uchida compared the period before the onset of rheumatoid arthritis to the period during involvement with the disease. Half of their female rheumatoid arthritis patients reported that they had decreased desire, decreased orgasms, and decreased frequency of intercourse.

Kraaimaat and associates sent a questionnaire to 500 arthritis impaired patients, to which 362 responded, and 220 of the respondents lived with a spouse. In this group of 220, there were 102 men and 118 women. They reported that rheumatoid arthritis almost never intruded into their marital relationship in 37% of men and 30% of women, it was sometimes intrusive in 32% of men and 34% of women, and almost always intrusive in 30% of men and 36% of women. This is a remarkably even spread between all of the options and between men and women.

Four intruding factors

The difficulties causing the intrusion of rheumatoid arthritis on sex were due to four factors: 1) difficulties with mobility or involvement of the lower extremities; 2) difficulties with self-care or involvement of the upper extremities; 3) depression; and 4) spousal criticism. Other factors mentioned by these patients were pain, fatigue, and social isolation.

In a study by Yoshino and Uchida entitled "Sexual problems in women with rheumatoid arthritis," 91 women answered a questionnaire regarding sexual problems. Fifty percent reported diminished desire, and reduced frequency to less than three times a month in 60%. Rheumatoid arthritis symptoms were worse the next day in 4% and more than 50% of them had joint pain during intercourse. Limited mobility interfered with sex when there was hip or knee involvement. In more than 60%, the patient and the husband were both dissatisfied with their sexual relationship. The relationship had deteriorated in about 10%, and improved in about 8%.

Sexual quality of life in arthritis

A study, "Sexual quality of life of patients with arthritis compared to arthritis-free controls," was reported by Blake and associates. They interviewed 169 patients. Rheumatoid arthritis had been diagnosed in 128 among whom 68% were early in the course of the disease and 32% had advanced disease. Osteoarthritis was the pattern in 38 patients. This involved knee in 15, hip in 3, spine in 9, hands in 6, and neck in 3. Five patients had ankylosing spondylitis. Controls were arthritis-free but pair-matched for age and gender. Of the arthritis patients, 36% were unsatisfied with sexual adjustment, compared to 39% of controls. Of the arthritis patients, 35% were satisfied with their sexual relationship, compared to 33% of controls. Fifteen percent were inactive sexually, but satisfied, compared with 17% of the controls. Thirty-one percent were anxious about their sexual performance, compared to 39% of the controls.

Blake also reviewed the causes of sexual dissatisfaction. In rheumatoid arthritis, 39% of women and 66% of men attributed their sexual dissatisfaction to pain, stiffness, and fatigue. This compared with 9% of the controls. Nineteen percent of the women and 12% of the men with rheumatoid arthritis felt unattractive compared to 18% of women and 8% of men in the control group.

Sexuality and chronic illness

Psychiatrist Thomas N. Wise, M.D., in a paper entitled "Sexuality and chronic illness," describes a 28-year-old woman who was seriously ill with systemic lupus erythematosus and associated renal failure. She had a long and stormy course in the Intensive Care Unit, but recovered, going through rehab treatment and ultimately returning home to her husband. When she got home she had an increased desire for sexual relations, but her husband made no attempt. She felt excluded and unworthy, and fortunately, at that point they sought counseling.

The counseling revealed that the husband was being protective, fearing he might hurt her. With that information they resumed sexual activity with a full response. This story emphasizes the profound need for the interpersonal relationship imparted by sex. Desire for sex had persisted in spite of the prolonged and devastating period of illness.

Dr. Wise points out that sexual dysfunction occurs in physically ill individuals in three capacities: the psychological capacity, the capacity for organic performance, and the capacity for organic enjoyment.

Emotional withdrawal is a result of feeling ill. Associated with it are lack of energy, fatigue due the disease, and fatigue due to pain. Pain restricts the ability of the patient to reach out emotionally. It saps one's energy and impairs physical ability to participate socially. This leads to social deprivation, and that in turn leads to loss of interest in activities. This develops into a loss of self esteem. It is complicated by the effect of medications. Emotional withdrawal is both cause and effect of fatigue, pain, and social deprivation.

Social and sexual interplay energizes

Happy social interplay is energizing. It distracts the perception of pain, and enhances the sense of self esteem. Sexual interplay is the most intimate and meaningful of social interplay. It is the most powerful antidote for the de-energizing loss of self esteem.

The capacity for organic performance is impacted by pain and loss of motion. Consider different positions and methods of providing sexual pleasure to your partner. It matters greatly that there is the comforting interpersonal communion.

The capacity for organic enjoyment is impaired by the loss of self-esteem, physical difficulties, and pain. The best support is a loving, caring sexual embrace frequently practiced.

Most medications used for treating arthritis have no impact on sexual capacity. The nonsteroidal anti-inflammatory drugs, including aspirin, ibuprofen, naproxen, and the newer COX-2 inhibitors such as celecoxib, rofecoxib, and valdecoxib, ease pain without affecting sexual capacity.

Morning sex

The time of day is important. Morning stiffness and evening fatigue are impediments. The man experiencing a testosterone surge in the morning may be better able to perform sexually at that time of day. A wife with arthritis may be too stiff in the morning. It is typical for the patient with arthritis to have an increased level of fatigue and, depending on disease activity, this occurs earlier and earlier in the evening. One may consider love in the afternoon.

The reactions of the spouse to the patient's pain and the importance of spousal support were reviewed in a number of studies. Kraaimaat, in a paper entitled "Association of social support and the spouse's reaction to psychological distress in male and female patients with rheumatoid arthritis," noted that pain and spousal criticism were important in both men and women, and were significantly associated with debility from depression and anxiety. Social support reduced psychological distress, but patients benefited clearly from spousal support.

Relationships and coping with chronic pain

Janice Snelling reported the effect of chronic pain on the family unit in a study of 18 patients with chronic pain and their partners, and one adult child of these patients. Two main variables emerged: *social relationships* and *coping techniques*.

The elements and types of social relationships that were affected were the marital partnership, sexual activity, contact with friends and relatives, and role changes. Chronic pain caused social isolation and role tension, marital conflict, and reduced sexual activity. Other family members had feelings of anger, resentment, and despondency.

Coping effectiveness in the patient determined the extent to which chronic pain negatively affected the partner or family. Chronic pain changes the marital partnership from one of equality to a dependent/dominant relationship. Chronic pain impinges on the sexual relationship. It can cause stress and arguments, and feelings can deteriorate to repugnance and withdrawal.

Family roles and feelings

Chronic pain changes roles in the family. Duties are loaded on the partner. The partner feels cheated and abused, or the partner may sacrifice growth at work due to increased demands at home. Chronic pain produces frustration, which leads to irritability. Because of the irritability, the children are yelled at and neglected, and the patient becomes increasingly isolated from friends and social outlets.

Mental problems and arthritis

Mental problems in rheumatoid arthritis were discussed in an editorial in the British Medical Journal under the title "Psychogenic factors can cause deterioration." The author noted that an emotional upset can precipitate an exacerbation of rheumatoid arthritis. Examples given of emotional upset were the emotional responses to the death of a loved one, the waywardness of an adolescent child, or the infidelity of a spouse. Indeed, the reassuring effect of intimacy is very important.

H.L.F. Currey sent a questionnaire to 121 married patients with osteoarthritis. All of them were under age 61, and all of them had prior hip surgery for osteoarthritis. Eighty one of them (67%) had sexual difficulty due to the arthritis. This was usually caused by pain and stiffness, and not due to loss of libido, but it was the cause of marital unhappiness in about a fourth of them.

"Spousal criticism and support, and their association with coping and psychological adjustment among women with rheumatoid arthritis," is the title of a paper by Doctors Mann and Zautra. They identify the family environment as a key to the adaptation of the patient. Criticisms of the spouse were associated with maladaptive coping. Social support was helpful, criticism harmful. Self-esteem was most likely to be harmed by spousal criticism. What husbands often criticized were the limitations imposed by the rheumatoid arthritis on social activities, recreational activities, and sexual activities. They did not complain as much about feeling burdened.

Marital conflict and interaction

In "The role of pain behaviors in the modulation of marital conflict in chronic pain couples," a study by Schwartz, et al, chronic-pain patients and their spouses responded to marital conflict with increased pain behavior. The spouse's negative feelings about the patient's pain relate to the perception that the pain behavior is in response to marital conflict. The spouses who feel more negative about the patient's pain are more likely to react punitively. The spouse's punitive responses to the patient's pain behavior elevate the pain to higher intensity and greater psychosocial and functional impairment.

Marital satisfaction was inversely related to feelings of isolation and depression, and enhanced by happiness and psychological well-being. This is discussed in a paper, "Marital interaction in the health and well-being of spouses," by Schmoldt et al. This paper lists the four qualities of marital interaction as consisting of cohesion, consensus, companionship, and cooperation.

Cohesion, consensus, companionship, and cooperation

Cohesion is defined as attachment, togetherness, and bonding. *Consensus* means shared beliefs, attitudes, and values. *Companionship* describes joint activities of husband and wife. *Cooperation* is the ability to collaborate. Schmoldt's study consisted of interviews from 1529 families in the Northwest Kaiser program centered in Portland, Oregon. There were 1004 married couples interviewed, and husband and wife were each interviewed separately. They found that the marital interaction was related to health and well-being, particularly as it involved cooperation, companionship, and cohesion, but not consensus. Social support was found to be of major importance in managing social tension. Without successful tension management, stress results. Marital interaction is a particularly important source of social support and protection from a diminished sense of well-being.

Sexual problems in arthritis and spondylitis

In a paper entitled "Sexual problems in rheumatoid arthritis and ankylosing spondylitis," Elst described a study of 188 patients who were compared to 475 controls. Fifty men and 16 women had ankylosing spondylitis, 32 men and 90 women had rheumatoid arthritis, and there were 236 men and 239 women in the control group. A questionnaire was followed by an interview. The questionnaire included several questions posed as statements with a range of possible answers, among them:

> It is difficult for me to get around:

> Most of the time, Often, Now and then, Seldom, Never

> I enjoy having sexual intercourse with my partner:
>
> Enjoy very much, much, a little, don't enjoy, don't enjoy at all.

The questionnaires were scored and compared to controls. Patients with ankylosing spondylitis had scores similar to those of the controls. With rheumatoid arthritis, enjoyment was less in both men and women, foreplay was shorter for both men and women, orgasm intensity was unchanged in both men and women, and frequency of intercourse was unchanged for both men and women. Greater disease severity scores were associated with less sexual motivation and lower disease severity scores correlated with greater sexual motivation. A lower sedimentation rate, which is a laboratory measure that indicates decreased disease inflammatory activity, was associated with greater sexual motivation. Fatigue and pain had inhibiting effects on desire.

During the interview portion of this study by Elst, a picture of couples in five coital positions was shown, and the questions asked were: "Which is the most satisfying," and "Which is the least painful." The traditional man-on-top position was the most satisfying in 42 percent, and the least painful in 33 percent. Of the other four positions, whichever position was selected as the one most satisfying was also judged most frequently to be the least painful.

In another study, a questionnaire concerning sexual problems was given to 112 female rheumatoid arthritis patients. Replies were collected from 91 of these patients, and reported by Drs. Yoshino and Uchida. More than half of the women had experienced a diminished desire for sexual relationships since the onset of their illness. Nearly 60% reported that the frequency of intercourse was less than three times a month. The symptoms of arthritis were worse on the day following intercourse in only 4%. Improvement in arthritis symptoms was not addressed.

There was an aggravation of joint symptoms, occurring only sometimes in 18%, and here, half reported joint pain during intercourse. Limitations in joint mobility interfered with intercourse in 12 patients with hip arthritis and in 6 out of 8 with knee-joint involvement.

My perspective

Arthritis impacts our sexuality in many ways. The physical obstructions seem fairly obvious, but they can be overcome. The emotional effects are both less obvious and more difficult to overcome. They impede our ability to do the stuff of normal, healthy living. We need to understand these impediments and do something about them. Partners in our lives are an important source of understanding and support, and negative attitudes exhibited by them contribute to the emotional impact of arthritis. In fact, loving healthy sexual interplay, with or without coitus, can improve the arthritis that impacts our sexuality. And that is the subject of the next chapter.

17

The Effect of Sex on Arthritis

To understand how sex relates to arthritis we need to know about the roles played by the brain and the psyche, the immune system, and hormones. This combines the fields of psychology, neurology, immunology, and endocrinology. The study of the profound and complex inter-relationships between these systems reveals that the brain is the central source of control. The immune system and the endocrine system are the combined systems of defense and health maintenance. Various types of stress serve to signal different responses in all of these systems.

Stress

There are two basic kinds of stress, acute and chronic. Subdivided under acute stress, there is good and bad stress. About 20 years ago, the therapeutic community coined a word for good stress that never made it into dictionaries, "eustress." Eustress means that a stressful event creates a beneficial change in the body, instead of creating a harmful change, which is what "distress" does. Therefore, even if a change is stressful, it isn't perceived as bad. The individual thrives on the change even if the change is perceived as an inconvenience, and consequently there is no illness. Distress is the body's violent reaction to change causing harmful effects such as mental or physical illness.

Therefore, stress, as a broad term, denotes a stimulus that affects the body, but gets different responses depending on how one perceives the stressor. For example, a wedding is stressful, but also causes joy; the birth of a child is stressful, but is also a blessing. Loss of a job is stressful and distressing; death is stressful and distressing, but possibly perceived differently by those affected. For example, family members whose loved one died after a long and difficult illness may feel relief and/or bereavement. Or a classic of-two-minds event: A one-car accident totals your old junker, so now you *have* to buy the new car you have saved for.

Acute eustress is good. It stimulates the mind, the central nervous system, the immune system, and the endocrine system to protect and promote mental and physical well-being. Chronic stress is damaging. Having arthritis is a chronic stressful experience.

Sex as eustress

Like exercise, healthy, loving, mutual sex is a good stressor. It is a source of relaxation and emotional support, provides involvement and engagement, improves positive affect and reduces negative affect. It reduces stress reactivity and improves coping ability. It also stimulates secretion of the hormones oxytocin and prolactin, and prolactin in turn enhances normal immune reactivity.

The interrelationship of pain, stress, and health is reviewed in an excellent article by David E. Yocum,

M.D., and his associates. Both pain and stress are ultimately related through the central nervous system by mechanisms that result in a significant amount of interaction on several levels. Both acute and chronic pain result in increased stress. A feedback loop may then develop that intensifies the pain. Stress and pain are complex. They share pathways in the central nervous system, the endocrine system, and the immune system, with many interconnections and interrelationships. Therapies that improve psychological health and function can change pain and change outcomes.

HPA and SAM systems respond to stress

Stress stimulates the brain, activating the hypothalamus, and that in turn activates the pituitary and adrenal glands. That is the hypothalamic-pituitary-adrenal system (HPA). It also activates the sympathoadrenomedullary (SAM) system.

The HPA system starts with the release of corticotrophin releasing hormone (CRH) from the hypothalamus. In turn, it tells the pituitary gland to release adrenocortico-trophic hormone (ACTH), and this in turn tells the adrenal cortex to release the corticosteroids (cortisone) which suppress the immune system. The SAM system wires you for action. It releases epinephrine (adrenalin) and norepinephrine (noradrenalin), substances which stimulate your immune system. Together both systems prepare you for the "fight or flight" response.

Prolactin

The pituitary gland also releases prolactin. This is the hormone that induces milk production and release in nursing mothers. Prolactin is also very important in maintaining and supporting our ability to mount an immune response. Hypophysectomy, the removal of the pituitary gland (in rats), causes prolactin levels to fall, and both antibody and cellular immunity decrease. This can be reversed by prolactin administration.

Prolactin administration produces an increase in the messenger protein Interleukin-2, which is also known as a growth factor for activated immune system T cells. It promotes cloning of these cells, thereby promoting the body's immune defenses. It is noteworthy that both the T lymphocytes, which are responsible for cellular immunity, and the B lymphocytes, that produce antibodies, have surface receptors for prolactin. In other words, the lymphocytes that are responsible for defending us against invading organisms or alien proteins respond to prolactin and are impaired in its absence. So, briefly, the good stressors stimulate increased corticosteroids, increased prolactin, and an increased ratio of corticosteroids to prolactin.

Corticosteroids and the immune response

Immunologically, corticosteroids decrease the ability of the immune lymphocytes to migrate through the tissues, and enhance the breakdown of lymphocytes. It reduces the circulating numbers of monocytes and macrophages, which are the cells that function as major controlling centers for the immune system. The macrophages capture the invading organisms, partially digest them into smaller pieces, and display them for the lymphocytes to respond. Corticosteroids decrease the ability of these macrophages to present antigen to the lymphocytes.

The overall effect of stress on the host is complex, and dependent not only on the type and intensity of the stressor, but also on the physiologic response of the host at several levels. This complex interaction between the psychology, neurology, endocrinology, and immunology as it relates to autoimmune disease has been under intense study, and is still being defined as understanding grows.

Increased prolactin levels have been reported in rheumatoid arthritis and systemic lupus erythematosus. Usually this would be protective. Prolactin stimulates the cloning of lymphocytes. When a lymphocyte finds an invading enemy, a bacterium or virus for example, it clones itself. This is as if a lone soldier on the front, once stimulated could clone himself into a whole army, specialized to fight this particular invader. Prolactin promotes that cloning.

In a study of 10 rheumatoid arthritis patients and five controls, Jorgensen noted that basal ACTH and prolactin levels were similar in both. Corticotrophin releasing hormone stimulation increased ACTH and beta endorphin in the rheumatic patients. In other words, stress evoked release of the pain reliever beta-endorphin. Stimulation of another hypothalamic hormone, thyroid releasing hormone, (TRH) produced increased Prolactin in rheumatoid arthritis. Basal beta endorphin levels were elevated in rheumatoid arthritis, and the response increased after corticotrophin-releasing hormone. Comparison to controls demonstrated that this was related to rheumatoid arthritis and was not a normal response. This means that in rheumatoid arthritis, our stress response provides protective and pain-relieving effects. Remember that sex is a healthy stressor.

Stress studies

Manfred Schedlowski and his associates described the effects of acute stress during a parachute jump. Hormonal responses were studied in 23 military parachute jumpers. Twelve were experienced and 11 were inexperienced parachuters. Each subject performed two jumps. Prior to and immediately after each jump, blood samples were drawn and analyzed for cortisol, prolactin, thyrotropin, somatotropin, and leuteinizing hormone. There was a significant increase in cortisol, prolactin, and thyroid stimulating hormones after both jumps, and in both groups. There were no alterations in the somatotropic hormone or leuteinizing hormone. Stress induced hormonal changes were not affected by prior jump experience. There was no association between the endocrine variables and anxiety scores.

Beta-endorphin, but not substance P, is increased by acute stress in humans. Beta-endorphins are the natural endogenous opioids or painkillers. Substance P is a peptide (protein piece) that transmits pain in the spinal cord. Manfred Schedlowski and associates tested 47 inexperienced tandem parachuters and obtained blood two hours before, immediately after, and one hour after a parachute jump. They measured plasma concentrations of beta-endorphin and substance P. The substance P concentrations appeared to be unaffected by jump stress, but there was a transient, though insignificant, increase in the beta-endorphin levels immediately after jumping. Subjects in a higher anxiety state at the point of jumping displayed higher substance P values at all three time points compared to the low anxiety jumpers.

In a study by Tillman and associates, prolactin secretion was elevated following an orgasm and remained elevated for substantial time afterwards, but it was unchanged following sexual arousal without orgasm. They con-cluded that this was probably a form of feedback control responsible for the reduction of libido and gonadal function following orgasm.

The link between stress and disease activity

In a study of 41 women with established rheumatoid arthritis, Zautra, et al. found an association between daily stressors and disease activity. At baseline, circulating levels of prolactin and peripheral blood CD4 to CD8 T-cell ratios were found to be higher in rheumatoid arthritis than in osteoarthritis. However, the ratio of peripheral corticosteroids to prolactin was lower in rheumatoid arthritis. These studies begin to unravel the relationship between stress and neuroendocrine and immune function. One might expect that certain types of good stressors could lead to an increased corticosteroid-to-prolactin ratio, resulting in immunosuppression and less rheumatoid disease activity. The proposed immune effects would be a decrease in the ratio of CD4 to CD8 lymphocytes with activation of the CD8 cells. To investigate this, 20 postmenopausal women with established erosive and moderately active rheumatoid arthritis were chosen to take part in a week-long program at a health spa, the Canyon Ranch.

The study of these women is described in the paper by Dr. Yocum. The Canyon Ranch spa has a life-enhancement center designed to accommodate moderately disabled individuals. The study individuals were merged with another 20 individuals with various forms of arthritis who were not being evaluated. The program included daily lectures by non-medical individuals on the cause, pathogenesis, and treatment of arthritis and pain. Both standard and alternative methods of treatment were discussed. In addition, all of the people participating were involved in daily pool exercise or other non-weight-bearing exercise, a diet low in fat and daily programs of yoga, tai chi, and other exercises.

One week prior to the initiation of the program, all of the participants underwent laboratory stress reactivity testing during which blood was taken for hormone levels. Heart rate and blood pressure data were collected throughout the program. Tests of immune function, including mononuclear cell studies, lymphocyte studies, and the ability of the cells to respond to antigens and to proliferate were evaluated. Two weeks after the program, study individuals underwent repeat stress reactivity and immune testing. Throughout the study the subjects answered a variety of questionnaires related to depression, optimism, and stress.

One week after their stay at the Canyon Ranch spa there were significant increases in both corticosteroids and prolactin, and an increase in the corticosteroid-to-prolactin ratio in those patients with the highest rheumatoid disease activity. Immunologically, the CD4 helper T-cells decreased, and the CD8 killer T-cells increased. Psychological measures revealed that the Canyon Ranch experience resulted in a significant increase in positive affect scores, and a significant reduction in negative affect scores. Stress reactivity to laboratory stress testing was measured by heart rate, and this was significantly decreased after the Canyon Ranch intervention. The psychological tests documented decreased stress reactivity and increased coping skills. Twelve weeks after the spa program, only the coping skills remained significantly improved. Those subjects with the greatest disease activity appeared to be more reactive to the laboratory stressors. Since there was no comparison or control group, these results must be interpreted with caution.

Exercise and stress reduction

In another study, Cornett and Yocum and their associates also employed a Canyon-Ranch-like program with emphasis on exercise and stress reduction. The program ran for four weeks, with arthritis participants meeting three times a week for three hours each time. These patients had rheumatoid arthritis and/or osteoarthritis. The three-hour meetings incorporated an aquatic exercise regimen with a one-to-two hour lecture. The participants completed questionnaires designed to measure physical functioning, coping techniques, and social support at the beginning of the program, and at four weeks, three months, and six months after beginning the program.

At four weeks and at three months, participants noted behavioral changes such as deep breathing and relaxation had resulted in significantly enhanced pain coping mechanisms. There was a trend toward decreased pain and stiffness. No hormone levels or immune-function studies were measured in this study. The data suggest that exercise and stress reduction led to enhanced ability to deal with pain.

The link between pain and stress

Dr. Yocum emphasized that stress and pain mechanisms are complex and share many central nervous system pathways. Both are critical issues for patients with arthritis. The link between stress and neuro-endocrine-immune functions suggests that improved psychological and metabolic function could significantly change pain and improve the outcome for patients with arthritis. Consequently, programs using alternative therapies such as tai chi and meditation, in combination with traditional medications, appear to be beneficial in patients with arthritis. These patients appear to live better lives, and they have better long-term outcomes.

In "Chronic life stress alters sympathetic neuroendocrine and immune responsivity to an acute psychological stressor in humans," a study by J.L. Pike and associates compared 12 men with chronic life stress to 11 men without chronic life stress. They subjected the men to a laboratory stressor (mental arithmetic) and compared that to a nonstressful video control. They found that acute psychological stress caused subjective distress, accompanied by an increase in epinephrine and norepinephrine, increased beta endorphin release, increased ACTH and corticosteroid release, and a redistribution of NK natural killer immune cells into the peripheral circulation.

Vaccination to flu virus and hepatitis B virus in 32 people, caregivers of patients with Alzheimer's disease, was investigated by Dr. Glaser and associates. The caregivers had a significantly reduced response to vaccination. In a second study, 48 medical students were studied following hepatitis B vaccination. Those students who had greater social support and less anxiety and stress responded more vigorously to the vaccine.

Pawlak, et al, attempted to determine whether lupus patients differ from healthy controls in their response to stress. They analyzed heart rate, blood pressure, epinephrine and nor epinephrine concentration, lymphocyte subpopulations, NK natural killer cell activity, and the expression of receptors on peripheral blood monocytes for beta adrenergic agents before, immediately after, and one hour after a public speaking task. Participants included 15 lupus patients and 15 healthy subjects. Both groups demonstrated similar psychological, cardiovascular, and neuroendocrine responses to acute stress. In both groups, the natural killer cell numbers transiently increased after stress exposure but there was a significantly less pronounced change in the lupus patients. The NK natural killer cell activity increased in healthy controls, but not in lupus patients. The number of Beta-2 adrenoreceptors on the peripheral blood monocytes significantly increased only in the healthy subjects after stress, but not in the lupus patients.

Exton, Schedlowski, et al, found that orgasm by masturbation in women induced elevations in cardiovascular parameters such as blood pressure and pulse, as well as in levels of plasma epinephrine, and nor-epinephrine. Plasma prolactin substantially increased after orgasm, and remained elevated 60 minutes after sexual arousal. Sexual arousal also produced small increases in plasma LH (leuteinizing hormone) and testosterone concentrations. In contrast, plasma concentrations of corticosteroids, FSH (follicle stimulating hormone), beta endorphin, progesterone, and estradiol were unaffected by orgasm. They concluded that sexual arousal and orgasm produce a distinct pattern of neuroendocrine alterations in women, primarily inducing a long-lasting elevation in plasma prolactin concentrations. These results concur with those observed in men, suggesting that prolactin is an endocrine marker of sexual arousal and orgasm.

Oxytocin

Oxytocin is a neurohormone that is secreted and released by the pituitary gland, and is increased during orgasm in both men and women. It plays a key role in initiating delivery of a baby. It is also key in animals in the initiation of maternal behavior and the formation of adult pair bonds. Social stimuli are thought to induce oxytocin release, and thus make positive social contact more rewarding.

In a paper entitled "Preliminary research on plasma oxytocin," R.A. Turner reported that oxytocin levels increased in association with massage and with positive emotion, but decreased in relation to sad emotion. In this study, 25 normal adult women were given psychological imagery tasks and completed questionnaires on attachment and interpersonal problems. Blood samples were obtained by indwelling intravenous catheters before, during, and after three interventions in which they were given massage, positive emotion stimuli, and negative emotion stimuli.

Increased oxytocin levels were associated with massage and with positive emotion, but sad emotion decreased the oxytocin levels. Those who showed increased oxytocin with massage and positive emotion, but failed to decrease oxytocin levels during negative emotion were less likely to report interpersonal problems associated with intrusiveness. They also had less anxiety in close relationships. Women who were in couple relationships had greater increases in oxytocin in response to positive emotion. Serum oxytocin levels were significantly increased after orgasm in 12 healthy women described by Blaicher and associates.

Uvnas-Moberg published a study that shows that oxytocin reduces pain by producing an increased endogenous opioid release. In animal studies, oxytocin injections were repeated over a five-day period in both male and female animals. Tail flick tests demonstrated that oxytocin produced a reduction in pain. Blood pressure decreased 10 to 20 mm Hg, Corticosteroids and insulin levels increased. The healing rate of wounds also improved.

Naloxone blocks the effects of opioids. The reduced response to painful stimuli caused by oxytocin is inhibited by naloxone. Murphy et al investigated the effect of naloxone on plasma oxytocin levels during sexual activity in eight men. Following a double blind, two period, crossover design, they showed that plasma oxytocin rose to 362% of baseline values at orgasm after placebo administration, but there was no increase when naloxone had been given. Oxytocin enhances the level of subjective arousal and pleasure at orgasm in men. Blocking opioid receptors with naloxone inhibited sexual arousal and pleasure. These findings are evidence that oxytocin has an endorphin-like effect, or alternatively, that endorphins play a role in the human sexual response. Either way, the release of oxytocin during the sexual response has pain-relieving and wound-healing benefits. In brief, sex releases oxytocin that has significant opioid based pain relieving effects.

Carmichael, et al, reported a study of 13 women and 12 men in which each subject completed two or more tasks of self-stimulation while the investigators were monitoring blood pressure along with anal electromyography and anal plethysmography to five minutes beyond orgasm. The blood samples were obtained continuously for oxytocin levels. In addition, systolic blood pressure was recorded and the anal electromyography and anal plethysmography measured muscular contractions. All of these correlated highly with the intensity of orgasm both prior to and during orgasm. The number of anal contractions and the duration of orgasm were highly correlated. But, increased oxytocin levels correlated with subjective orgasm intensity only in multiorgasmic women.

Dr. Dean Edell, in his radio broadcast and on his web site, www.HealthCentral.com interviewed Dr. Rebecca Turner of UC San Francisco. Dr. Turner reported that women had higher oxytocin levels when they were in a close relationship, during positive emotional states, and when they were more secure in their relationships. Women who were not in a relationship had lower oxytocin levels and more difficulty with emotional openness. In the more secure subjects, the higher levels of oxytocin seemed in turn to reinforce their bond with their partners.

Basal ACTH and prolactin levels were similar in ten rheumatoid arthritis patients and five controls in a study reported by Jorgensen but beta endorphin was increased in the rheumatic patients. TRH (thyroid releasing hormone) stimulation produced increased prolactin in these people with rheumatoid arthritis. Basal beta endorphin levels were elevated in rheumatoid arthritis, and the response after administration of corticotrophin releasing hormone (CRH) was increased in comparison to controls

My perspective

The complexity of the psycho-neuro-immuno-endocrinology system is astounding, even to me after more than 40 years of study. But it is so very real, and so very important in life and in health. The recognition of the role of stress, both bad stress and eustress opens the door to understanding how sex can be beneficial.

Outstanding among the many fascinating and important insights are those relating to the role of prolactin and oxytocin. Prolactin enhances our self-defense system, the immune system. It is notable especially for its ability to stimulate cloning of lymphocytes. While rheumatoid arthritis and related diseases involve wayward immune responses, we still need an intact immune system. This is where the new biological remission inducing drugs are so exciting and valuable. They are like laser guided missiles in that they attack only one specific target, cutting through all the other processes involved in our self-defense and impact only the one doing harm. Prolactin, which is increased during and after sexual stimulation, supports the normal functioning of immunity.

Oxytocin, also pain relieving, is released during a sexual response. It works by the same mechanisms that make morphine effective. Both prolactin and oxytocin are prominent products of our sexual responses. Sex, healthy, safe, loving sex, provides emotional, psychological and physical-hormonal benefits for people with arthritis.

18

The Benefits of Alcohol

Moderate and appropriate use of alcohol can benefit people with arthritis. Patients with arthritis have an increased risk of atherosclerosis and coronary artery disease. Light to moderate alcohol consumption reduces insulin resistance, which inhibits atherosclerosis. It also inhibits platelet clotting that starts the occlusive plug that ultimately blocks the flow of blood in a damaged coronary artery. Alcohol scavenges the radicals of oxygen and nitrogen that oxidize low density cholesterol deposits that are the core of the atherosclerotic process.

In addition, the oxidative effects of reactive oxygen and nitrogen radicals play an important role in the inflammation of arthritis. And, alcohol scavenges and deactivates these radicals in the inflamed joints. As I stated at the beginning of this book, those who are recovering alcoholics, and those who do not want to drink alcohol, should not do so. Drinking alcohol in this case is an option, a complementary and alternative therapy, and is not essential for every person.

Insulin and cholesterol

In a study of 87 patients with rheumatoid arthritis in South Africa, nearly a third had insulin resistance, a condition that predisposes people to hardened arteries. Seventy percent had abnormal cholesterol levels. Family histories revealed that the incidence of premature coronary artery disease was more than three times that of a control group without arthritis.

Between 1964 and 1995, coronary artery disease was the most frequent cause of death in rheumatoid arthritis patients in Sweden. Records of 46,917 rheumatoid arthritis patients were reviewed and compared to the population at large. Those patients whose arthritis was first diagnosed between the ages of 20 and 39 years had a five fold increased risk of coronary death. After 1975, there was a decrease in the mortality rate among these patients, which was attributed to better access to rheumatologic care.

Myocardial infarction and congestive heart failure

In another study, 450 patients with rheumatoid arthritis were compared to age and sex-matched controls. Myocardial infarction and congestive heart failure were 50% more frequent in patients with rheumatoid arthritis. The risk is greater in men than in women. Patients with psoriatic arthritis have higher than normal levels of LDL, "bad cholesterol," and low levels of HDL, "good cholesterol." Higher mortality rates are predictable by more severe levels of rheumatoid arthritis. Coronary artery disease occurs more frequently in women with either rheumatoid arthritis or systemic lupus. Part of the risk in lupus, but not all of it, is related to the anti-phospholipid syndrome, which is often a component of lupus. It involves antibodies that cause excessive clotting.

There is also up to a five fold increase in the incidence of myocardial infarction in rheumatoid arthritis. Deaths due to coronary artery disease were 3.6 times higher in rheumatoid arthritis than in the normal population and strokes occurred at least six times more frequently.

Arthritis and coronary artery disease

There are a number of reasons why coronary artery disease, stroke, and atherosclerosis may be increased in rheumatoid arthritis and related diseases like lupus. These reasons include the involvement of the endothelial internal lining cells of the blood vessels in the inflammatory process. These endothelial cells are part of the immune system, and the endothelial lining is reactive. When the cells are stimulated, they contribute significantly to the immune response and to inflammation. Vascular inflammation is one of the major mechanisms for producing atherosclerotic cholesterol plaques. Low-density lipid is deposited in the wall of the artery, at sites that are apparently directed by an inflammatory process in the vessel lining. This "bad-cholesterol" deposit then is oxidized by reactive oxygen radicals, which, in turn, attracts more inflammatory cells that invade the involved area of the blood vessel. That causes it to thicken, and subsequently to occlude (block) the blood vessel, leading to arterial occlusion and heart attack or stroke. Alcohol, as I said above, works as an antioxidant to help prevent this blockage.

Estrogen also promotes clotting, which may help explain why women with rheumatoid arthritis or lupus are more prone to coronary artery disease and stroke. In addition, patients with lupus may have abnormal antibodies that promote clotting. These include the anti-phospholipid and anti-cardiolipin antibodies and lupus anticoagulant. This increases the risk of clot formation.

WHAT ALCOHOL DOES FOR THE HEART

Alcohol is an anti-oxidant

- o Scavenges superoxide and nitric acid radicals.

- o Blocks oxidation of LDL cholesterol in the arteries.

- o Blocks formation of the plaque formation that plugs arteries.

C-Reactive Protein (CRP)

One valuable laboratory test that is a measure of disease activity in rheumatoid arthritis is the measurement of C - reactive protein (CRP), which is produced by the liver, and its production is stimulated by interleukin-6. Interleukin-6 is the third cytokine to be released in the immune reaction that characterizes rheumatoid arthritis, following TNF alpha, and then interleukin-1. If the CRP is elevated, it signifies increased rheumatoid disease activity. If it is decreasing, it indicates improvement. C - reactive protein is present in atherosclerotic plaques (the same kind of CRP that typifies the inflammation of rheumatoid arthritis), but not in the normal arterial wall. It binds to damaged tissues and to lipoproteins, the lipid deposits of atherosclerosis. It induces the expression of adhesion molecules and other cytokines in the endothelial cells. More than a marker of inflammation, CRP amplifies it. If the CRP is increased, the risk of atherosclerotic heart disease is increased.

Separate from rheumatoid arthritis then, CRP levels are elevated in coronary artery disease before a heart attack occurs. This is associated with a progressive increase in the risk of death from myocardial infarction. It occurs whether the CRP is secreted in response to rheumatoid arthritis or lupus, or in coronary artery disease without any associated arthritis.

Cholesterol deposits in the walls of the arteries do not explain all of the features of the atherosclerotic lesions. Smooth muscle cells proliferate and form scars that attempt to wall off the cholesterol deposits. This is accompanied by an inflammatory response. The way it works is this: the low density lipid (LDL cholesterol) deposited in the arterial wall becomes oxidized, largely by the action of superoxide radicals. These are released during an inflammatory reaction. When the immune cells react, one of the things they do is to make cytokines. These are proteins that carry messages or instructions to other cells. Among them are growth promoting factors. After the growth factors are released, they promote proliferation of smooth muscle cells and other inflammatory cells, like the monocytes that then invade the area. This invasion by immune system cells is a core development in the inflammation that occurs.

WHAT ALCOHOL DOES FOR ARTHRITIS

Alcohol is an antioxidant.

- Scavenges superoxide and nitric acid radicals.

- Blocks the inflammatory and destructive activity of the radicals

- Reduces pain, swelling and destructive activity in the joint.

- Reduces the increased risk of coronary artery disease in arthritis.

For the monocytes to invade the area, the arterial wall has to become "sticky." This occurs when adhesion molecules like vascular cell adhesion molecule-1 (VCAM-1) and intercellular adhesion molecule-1 (ICAM-1) and some other cytokines are released. The sticky artery lining cells attract or capture circulating monocytes and other inflammatory cells in the blood. When the monocytes are attached to the surface of the endothelial lining cells, they literally roll along like little balls until they come to the junction between two endothelial cells. Then the monocytes squeeze between these endothelial cells and migrate through the endothelial lining to become tissue macrophages. That process has been recorded with special microphotograpic methods in which one can watch the monocytes attach, roll and migrate beneath the endothelium. There they ingest lipid deposits to form foam cells. This is when the smooth muscle cells proliferate and get involved. The lesion then progresses from a fatty streak filled with oxidized LDL laden macrophages, to the more advanced fibrous plaque. If the monocytes are prevented from entering the arterial wall, atherosclerosis is inhibited.

Neoangiogenesis and alcohol

In arthritis, and after a heart attack, neoangiogenesis is stimulated. This is the process of forming new blood vessels. It is both a part of healing and repair in the heart, and a part of the inflammation of arthritis. It is one component of the swelling and proliferation of the invasive synovial tissue that digests and destroys cartilage and bone. The swollen tissue needs to grow its own blood supply. That is how it gets started. Alcohol helps inhibit neoangiogenesis.

Alcohol helps control the ravages of inflammation by scavenging destructive superoxide and nitric acid radicals. Oxygen forms radicals with an extra electron in its outer valence or orbit. These reactive oxygen species, and like them, reactive nitrogen species, are important products of inflammation and they have destructive power of their own. Alcohol deactivates these radicals. Compounds found in certain foods may be able to significantly bolster biological resistance against oxidants. Great interest centers on the possible protective value of a wide variety of plant-derived antioxidant compounds, particularly those from fruits and vegetables. Alcohol qualifies, both as a product of fruit and vegetables and as an antioxidant.

The "French Paradox"

A chart of Europe showing the geographic variations in the incidence of cardiovascular death led to the discovery of "the French Paradox." The northern countries had double or triple the cardiovascular death rate of those countries in the south. The pattern followed the intake of animal fat in the diet, except in France. "The French Paradox" is explained by the relative consumption of wine. Scotland, Finland, and the United States consume the least wine and have the most disease. Belgium, West Germany, and Austria consume more wine and have less disease. Switzerland, Italy, and France use the most wine and have the lowest rate of cardiovascular disease.

The oxygen paradox

Superoxide and nitric oxide molecules damage tissues by oxidizing them. "The oxygen paradox" was described and reviewed in an excellent article entitled "Oxidative Stress: The paradox of aerobic life," by K. J. Davies. The oxygen paradox states that higher aerobic organisms cannot exist without oxygen, yet oxygen is dangerous to their existence. This "dark side" of oxygen relates directly to the fact that each oxygen atom has one unpaired electron in its outer valence shell. Atomic ion oxygen is a free radical. The superoxide anion radical along with hydrogen peroxide and the extremely reactive hydroxyl radical are common products of life in an aerobic environment, and these agents are responsible for oxygen toxicity. To survive in such an unfriendly oxygen environment, living organisms need and generate or garner from their surroundings a variety of water and lipid soluble antioxidant compounds. A series of antioxidant enzymes, whose role is to intercept and inactivate reactive oxygen intermediates, is synthesized by all known aerobic organisms. Although extremely important, these antioxidant enzymes and compounds are not completely effective in preventing oxidative damage. To deal with the damage that does still occur, other natural enzymes are generated to protect proteins, lipids, and DNA.

Oxidative stress

In spite of antioxidant and repair mechanisms, oxidative damage remains an inescapable outcome of aerobic existence. In recent years, oxidative stress has been implicated in a wide variety of degenerative processes, diseases, and syndromes. These include mutation of cells, cell transformation in cancer; arteriosclerosis, heart attacks and strokes. Ischemia or lack of blood supply is followed by reperfusion (restoration of blood flow to an organ or tissue after blood supply has been cut off) injury once the flow of blood resumes and oxygen is carried to the area.

Reperfusion injury is the reaction to a build-up of superoxide radicals that are responsible for most of the damage to cardiac muscle during a heart attack. During the period of occlusion of the coronary artery, adequate oxygen is not available in the ischemic area. Oxygen radicals are generated when the vessel opens and perfusion is permitted. At this point, the superoxide radicals perfuse the heart muscle involved and cause the tissue damage.

Superoxide dismutase (SOD)

Superoxide dismutase, a natural enzyme, can protect the myocardium from this damage, but not if it is taken orally because our gastric juices digest it. Injections are needed early in the course of a heart attack, if it is available. But it is not available. The company that was developing it was disbanded after several episodes of management problems, and time ran out on the patent. The cost was prohibitive, too. The interesting tie-in to arthritis is that, injected into joints afflicted with osteoarthritis or rheumatoid arthritis, SOD provided long-lasting relief.

Chronic inflammatory diseases, like rheumatoid arthritis, lupus erythematosus, and psoriatic arthritis do involve reactive oxygen and nitrogen radicals in the tissues under attack. Here too, these radicals are destructive and contribute substantially to the damage being done. The superoxide radicals, hydrogen peroxide and nitric oxide, are produced by the inflammatory process and then are converted into the highly reactive hydroxyl radicals that react with almost all molecules in living cells. Suryaprabha demonstrated that superoxide and hydrogen peroxide are generated by peripheral white blood cells and significantly increased in rheumatoid arthritis and systemic lupus erythematosus. A study reported by J. Sung demonstrated that reactive oxygen production is increased in rheumatoid arthritis synovial (joint lining) cells, too. Interleukin-6 increases the production of oxygen radicals and it is one of the major products in the inflammatory process in rheumatoid arthritis. They examined the effects of methotrexate on the synthesis of interleukin-6 and on fibroblast-like synovial cells from the joint of a patient with rheumatoid arthritis. Under the influence of interleukin-6 the fibroblast-like cells proliferated and produced superoxide radicals. These cells were accompanied by inflammatory immune cells and new blood vessels. This mass of fibroblast-like synovial cells and immune and other inflammatory cells and new blood vessels grow into the joint. There they spread out over the cartilage and bone and digest them. This is how the damage is done. It was inhibited in the presence of methotrexate.

In rheumatoid arthritis, the inflammatory reaction in the synovial joint tissue is enhanced by the production of interleukin-6 with the subsequent generation of C -

reactive protein and reactive oxygen radicals. The same process occurs in atherosclerotic cardiovascular disease. Oxygen radicals are significant in both situations, and so is the ability of alcohol to deactivate these radicals.

In a report by J. C. Ruf the importance of platelet aggregation and atherothrombosis or clotting of the blood at the site of the atherosclerotic lesion is emphasized. Plasma high-density lipid is inversely correlated with coronary heart disease. In other words, high levels of HDL are protective. The protective effect of alcoholic beverages is certainly partly due to its ability to stimulate increased levels of HDL cholesterol. But it is also due, perhaps to the extent of 50%, to decreased platelet activity. The anti-platelet activity of wine is explained not only by the alcohol, but also by the poly-phenols in the wine with which red wines are richly endowed. These exert their effects by reducing production of prostaglandins that are involved in platelet aggregation and clotting. The phenolics in wine can reduce the increased platelet activity mediated by another reactive radical, nitric oxide. Wine phenolics also increase vitamin E levels while they decrease the oxidation of platelets submitted to oxidative stress. A rebound phenomenon of increased coagulability is observed after acute alcohol consumption, but not after wine consumption. This protection, afforded by wine, has been duplicated in animals with grape phenolics added to alcohol.

A study reported by Agewall, et al, entitled "Does a Glass of Red Wine Improve Endothelial Function?" examined the acute effects of red wine and de-alcoholized red wine. Drinking red wine caused arterial dilation and increased blood flow. These changes were not observed with de-alcoholized red wine and were therefore attributed directly to alcohol.

"Shaken, not stirred."

Trevithick, et al, published an article entitled "Shaken, Not Stirred: Bio Analytical Study of the Antioxidant Activities of Martinis." This was a reference to the film character James Bond's remark that he wanted his martinis "shaken, not stirred." That led to the study in which stirred and shaken martinis were assayed for their ability to quench luminescence. "Luminescence" is a measure of reactive oxygen activity. They showed that shaken martinis were more effective in deactivating hydrogen peroxide than the stirred variety, and both were more effective than gin or vermouth alone. The reason remains unclear. They explained that martinis are less well endowed with polyphenols than Sauvignon white wine or Scotch whiskey. They attributed 007's profound state of health to be due, at least in part, to compliant bartenders.

Purple grape juice improves endothelial function. A study designed to evaluate this demonstrated that short-term ingestion of purple grape juice improved flow-mediated vasodilation. In addition, the susceptibility of low-density lipid (LDL) particles to be oxidized was reduced.

The phenolics in wine can reduce platelet activity mediated by nitric oxide. Wine phenolics also increase vitamin E levels and they decrease the oxidation of platelets submitted to oxidative stress. A rebound phenomenon of increased coagulability was observed after acute alcohol consumption, but not after wine consumption. This protection, afforded by wine, has been duplicated in animals with grape phenolics added to alcohol.

Sex and alcohol

Like sex, alcohol has both biological and emotional benefits. Arthritis causes a whole series of reactions that impact your social life and your partner's. Psychosocial factors include depression, poor self-image, and social isolation, even in your own home. These elements, added to pain, fatigue, and apprehension, seriously affect your sexuality and the relationship between you and your partner. You may feel less attractive, or hold back because of concerns about pain. Deep down, arthritis may affect your ability to live and participate with those you love. Your partner might experience similar problems: fear of causing pain, sensing your apprehension and depression, and/or feeling rejected when you say you are too tired or not in the mood. Alcohol, appropriately enjoyed, can help ease the social elements.

A word of caution

Overdosing on alcohol to the point of inducing a hangover is a bad stressor and aggravates the symptoms you want to relieve. The symptoms of alcoholic hangover are caused by a combination of dehydration, hormonal alterations, dysregulated cytokine pathways, and direct toxic effects of alcohol. The physiologic effects include increased cardiac work and diffuse slowing of brain EEG activity.

The symptoms of hangover were reviewed and mechanisms discussed in an article published in *Annals of Internal Medicine*, June 2000. Jeffrey Wiese, M.D. and his associates had reviewed medical literature for the 33-year period from 1966 to 1999. Alcohol abuse and resulting hangover, they show, is a risk factor for cardiac death. Impaired alertness and decreased cognitive ability both carry an increased risk of accidents and endanger others. In addition, it produces social complications, like job loss and decreased productivity.

Moderate alcohol intake is defined variously. Most authorities allow two normal drinks per day for men and one for women. One liberal definition of moderate alcohol use allowed up to 3½ glasses of wine or three 12-ounce bottles of beer or three 1-ounce shots of 80 proof whiskey per day. More than that certainly is considered excessive. In 1979, 24% of all adults in the United States were reported as moderate drinkers, one third as light drinkers, the other third as abstainers, and 9% as heavy drinkers.

By the time you feel you are getting intoxicated, you've overdosed. Stop. Listen to your body. Women generally tolerate alcohol less well than men, because women are often smaller, metabolize alcohol differently, and respond to it more strongly. So be conservative. Also, don't make a habit of drinking every day. Vary the pattern. It only takes three weeks to make a habit and this habit is complicated by the dependency called addiction, which is a much higher mountain to overcome than a habit.

Benefiting from moderate consumption

Cynthia Baum-Baicker notes that moderate alcohol consumption reduces stress, tension, depression, and self-consciousness. It increases social interaction in the affective expression of happiness, conviviality, and euphoria. Low doses of alcohol have been found to improve certain types of cognitive performance, including problem solving and short-term memory. Cognitive abilities like these tend to be impaired in chronic systemic disease like systemic lupus and rheumatoid arthritis. This may be a direct effect of the disease in central nervous system lupus, or a secondary manifestation of the chronic fatigue that exists in most chronic inflammatory diseases. Regular moderate drinkers have less clinical depression than both abstainers and heavy drinkers, and alcohol in low and moderate doses has been effective in the treatment of psychiatric problems in geriatric patients.

Alcohol reduces the magnitude of the physiologic responses to stressful stimuli. This was demonstrated by recording electro dermal responses to loud sounds or to verbal stimuli and responses of cardiac rate and function to loud sounds before and after alcohol.

Alcohol may provide periods of relief from emotional tension from environmental stresses, and decreased depression and self-consciousness via alcohol's fear-reducing property. Low and moderate alcohol intake has also been reported to increase overall affective expression, happiness, euphoria, and pleasant, carefree feelings. However, one study correlated significantly drinking for stress relief with economic hardship, anxiety, low self-esteem, and a low sense of mastery.

The emotional responses of nonalcoholic subjects from the effects of moderate alcohol consumption varied with drinking patterns. Increased sexual and aggressive behavior was found in heavier drinkers. Women were more likely to experience positive general, social, and physical pleasure factors from moderate alcohol use. Men were most likely to experience an arousal of power and aggression, increased social assertiveness along with relaxation and reduction of tension. After modest doses of alcohol, drinkers experience effects that are largely due to natural expectations. That is, they stay "in character." Heavier intake causes more direct pharmacologic effects that are physiologically and psychologically damaging.

My perspective

For those who can't drink, or choose not to, other dietary regimens can help fight the cholesterol related cardiovascular problems that alcohol helps control. The benefits of moderate alcohol intake, and of wine in particular, include both psychological support and enhanced cardiovascular health. Alcohol scavenges reactive oxygen and nitrogen species, and this applies both to atherosclerosis and to the tissue damage that occurs in rheumatoid arthritis and lupus. It probably also holds true for osteoarthritis. Alcohol enhances insulin sensitivity, which reduces triglyceride levels and atherosclerosis, and increases high-density lipid levels that have a protective role against atherosclerosis. It promotes increased blood flow, and reduces platelet clotting, thereby inhibiting the starting mechanism of a coronary occlusion. These processes are important also in arthritic inflammatory processes in the joint.

While the benefits accruing from alcohol have been publicized for cardiovascular disease, they have not been recognized for arthritis until now. The role of reactive oxygen and nitrogen radicals in inflammation is well known, and the effect of alcohol is not restricted to the heart and blood vessels. Also, it is only recently that we have realized that the risk of atherosclerotic cardiovascular disease is increased in arthritis. This makes the importance of alcohol in arthritis more significant.

19

Enjoying Alcohol

A key to starting a romantic encounter is to set the mood. Wine and other alcoholic beverages can help. The benefits of gentle stroking and massage in promoting a recovery of your sexual relationship are like the benefits of alcohol. Use it for fun and relaxation. Use it as a way of sharing. Sharing a good wine is a classic way to relax and close out the stresses of life. Start by learning about wines. Discover your preferences. For those who already are experienced in wine selection, these suggestions may still bring up some fun ideas. For those who are novices, they should be at least as much fun.

If you can find a good wine bar in your neighborhood or town, ask them to set up a sampling of four good wines. You should be given a small serving, perhaps a half glass of each of four different wines to taste and compare. Start with four types of white wine: a sauvignon blanc, a dry chardonnay, an oaky chardonnay and a rich buttery chardonnay. Swirl each one in your glass and then hold it to your nose. Notice the fragrance. Do it again. Then take a sip and taste it in your mouth and again on the way down. What is the after taste? Before you taste the next one, have a bite of plain bread to clear your palate, and then perhaps some water before proceeding to the next glass. Take a bottle of your favorite wine home for another day.

Next time, try four red wines. Try a petit sirah, a pinot noir, a cabernet sauvignon and a merlot or a zinfandel. Explore over time the differences between different winemakers by comparing the same varietal prepared by different vintners. Compare California, New York, French, Italian and Australian wines. You can have a great time with this game. The best times though will be quietly at home together as part of a romantic moment. A favorite of mine is the Italian wine from Verona—Bolla Valpolicella.

A new twist on the wine tasting is called a wine blending party. Here, a wine expert or two set up a series of tables with the same three different wines on each. Perhaps a cabernet sauvignon, a merlot or a pinot noir and a white, perhaps a sauvignon blanc or a pinot blanc. Each table accommodates four or six participants. Empty demi-bottles are provided for each participant along with a self adhesive label and colored drawing pens. A paper listing the three varieties of wine is provided for each table. Each participant designs his or her own blend using all three of the wines provided. The percentage of each wine in your own blend is recorded at the time of mixing. Then, the partners at each table taste each other's blend, and select one as their product.

A name for the blended product and a label are created by the contestants at each table and applied to the demi-bottle with the blend chosen for submission. Finally, the wine experts taste the submitted blends and select the best. A prize of a bottle of wine is given to each member of the group with the best blend. A second prize for the best label is similarly awarded and a third prize goes to the group that showed the most "spirit." No fair getting a head start to build up a spirited euphoria. You can learn a lot about wines in this game and it's fun.

You can enjoy the tasting game with beer but blending has not been tried so far as I know. There is a wonderful variety of beers. International and national breweries and local microbreweries offer beers with widely varying flavors, colors and consistencies.

The comfort, relaxation, and social interplay that accompany good wine or cocktails are legendary. Alcohol, taken in moderation is effective in reducing stress. This is true both for the subjective sense of feeling less stress and for physiologic measures of the effect of stress. Alcohol increases your ability to express your thoughts and feelings and to communicate better. It enhances happiness, euphoria, conviviality, and pleasant and carefree feelings. Drinking for the pleasure of it should involve companionship. In turn, sharing wine or cocktails leads to improved communication, a feeling of togetherness, and it lends emotional warmth to the companionship.

If you are allergic to wine, are taking a medication that forbids drinking alcohol, if wine gives you a headache, or makes you feel depressed, you can be part of the social group and drink grape juice as an alternative that offers some but not all of the benefits offered by wine. Look for the growing variety of non-alcoholic grape juice substitutes for wine in your wine store or grocery store.

Learning about wine

Love by the Glass, written by Dorothy Gaiter and John Brecher, a couple who became full time wine writers for the *Wall Street Journals*' "Tastings" column, is a delightful story about their discovery of wine, and an education about different kinds of wine from around the world. Their book tells a charming story with a great deal of insight about how to enjoy wine, and includes descriptions of the individual characteristics of different wines from different wine makers. It is a good way to learn about the different types of wine. Some of their comments in the epilogue shed a little insight into the color of their book.

Another book worth reading for both beginners and experienced wine drinkers is *Pairing Wine And Food*, by Linda Johnson-Bell. This is an excellent description of the different kinds of wine, how to identify them, how to describe them, what to look for in them, how they relate to foods, how to use them, and how to enjoy them.

Another book you should know about whether you are a novice or an expert on wines is *Good Wine Guide 2002*, by Robert Joseph. This is an excellent presentation about wines, what they are, which ones are good, and where they come from. It's the best wine geography text I have seen. It includes maps that show the wine producing areas around the world, and it lists and describes the elements of wine tasting and the character of wines and a price range for each type. It is interesting reading and can be the basis for a wine tasting at home or at a wine cellar.

Another fun project, after you've done your homework and gotten some lessons at wine tastings, is to start a small wine cellar of your own. Wine should be selected for its ability to age well. White wines age poorly as a rule, although I have seen some good buttery and oaky chardonnay age with improvement for several years. Aging is best attempted with red wines. Red wines with body. Voluptuous reds. Buy a few bottles at a reasonable price, set them in the cellar and open one every six to twelve months …or longer if you're brave. I have been richly rewarded by this project. After you have one you like, well aged and beautifully matured, it can be an outstanding accompaniment to a beautiful dinner. And you would pay a great deal more to buy it after it has aged.

Be careful how you store your wine. Wine is best stored at a cool temperature. The basement may be good in winter. I had a room in the back of my garage where I installed an air conditioner. The walls were insulated with shelves of old books, and the weather cooperated to help me keep the temperature at about 60 degrees F. In the winter, the outside temperature kept it at about 50 degrees. That worked very well.

Keep your wine on its side, so the cork doesn't get dry, which would let air get in and allow the wine to oxidize into vinegar. Even if that happens, don't toss it out; use it in a stew. It will rarely get sour, but if it does, add a little sugar. Also, you can add herbs and a source of protein, like chicken wings or necks, or a beef bone. Then simmer that down to a thick gelatinous sauce, and use it in cooking. Wild duck poached in the wine and then served cold with the reduced wine sauce as a topping is delicious. Red wine is best but you can use white. If you want, add some port or sherry to the sauce before reducing it to a syrupy consistency. Serve individual portions dressed in the wine sauce, on a bed of shredded lettuce with a light olive oil vinaigrette and garnish it with dried cranberries plus a pickled crab-apple for a delicious lunch or first course.

My perspective

Food and wine are fun. Use grape juice or fruit juice if you don't want wine.

20

The Ultimate Alternative

Arthritis impacts sexuality adversely. In contrast, the emotional and biological benefits of sex and alcohol on arthritis are valuable in reducing the effects of arthritis. The biological effects of sex have been studied well, but not as well as they need to be. And they have not been viewed previously from the perspective of the eustress of a loving caring sexual relationship in the face of arthritis. Likewise, the biological health benefits of alcohol were identified for cardiovascular disease, but they apply as well to the inflammatory processes involved in arthritis. The benefits of sex and of alcohol for arthritis care are new concepts. They have always existed, but were not identified previously.

Arthritis' beginnings can be abrupt, but usually are gradual. The symptoms often are ignored and neglected until they become too pronounced and intrusive to deny. The pattern of initial awareness varies with different types of arthritis. It can be localized to one joint and limited to certain kinds of activities, or it can be generalized and diffuse, with pain and swelling involving many joints, accompanied by generalized symptoms like the morning stiffness so common to all.

The intrusion of arthritis on lifestyle and the emotional response to it vary considerably. Rheumatoid arthritis serves as a focal point for this discussion, but the principles apply to all kinds of arthritis, as well as to fibromyalgia and the other connective tissue diseases. Also, since rheumatoid arthritis occurs in women more frequently than in men, we have focused on women as the patients, but the obverse is equally applicable.

Morning stiffness is a generalized, but sometimes localized, feeling much like the stiffness common after a long automobile trip. Getting out of bed in the morning finds most of us a little stiff for the moment, but with arthritis, the stiffness is more pronounced and persists longer. It is associated with pain and usually involves more joints and muscles. This is so characteristic that it is used as a measure of disease activity. Its presence is a significant diagnostic criterion. If the stiffness doesn't last more than a few minutes, it is of doubtful diagnostic significance. If it lasts for five hours or more it is a sign of severe disease. Shortening of the duration of morning stiffness is a measure of improvement.

Testosterone levels run highest in the morning, so men tend to desire sex then, but the stiffness of muscles and joints intrudes. When women are the ones with morning stiffness, they are unlikely to feel responsive to sexual overtures. So men feel rejected, and after a while withdraw their morning ardor. That's the beginning.

Often the diagnosis of arthritis provokes general depression and produces a grieving process that manifests in denial and guilt, then anger, depression, and these emotions can cause serious loss of libido.

Fatigue is another hallmark of rheumatoid arthritis. The length of time from arising in the morning until the onset of fatigue is another valid measure of disease severity.

When the fatigue takes over at mid or late afternoon, there is no energy for evening activities. The family's after-school needs become a heavy burden, and there is neither energy nor desire for a sexual relationship.

Painful joints also play a significant role. Certain positions can be painful, depending on the joints that are involved. When you fear hurting your partner, or being hurt, sexual responsiveness is inhibited, followed by difficulty maintaining an erection or lack of lubrication. Arthritis imposes simple mechanical problems that dictate avoiding certain positions.

Anxiety, frustration, and depression about being ill with an unpredictable disease further intrude on the relationship. Fear of deformity adds to the emotional load. Once physical changes have occurred, she feels unattractive and withdraws further. He is clueless about her feelings unless they discuss them, and usually they don't.

No desire, no sex, and partners drift apart. He knows she hurts and is fearful of hurting her. She is fearful too, and lacking the energy, she doesn't care about finding comfortable positions and activities. Life goes on, but the warmth and support of an affectionate sexual relationship is lacking. You are depriving yourself of the much needed emotional and physiologic benefits of sex.

When you are first diagnosed with arthritis, you might think your life is over, but it's not. You need to learn new and different ways of doing the things you like to do. One day you decide you're not going to give in to it. You are going to have a life! This is where a loving, supportive relationship becomes most helpful. Depression is a result of the physical limitations that arthritis causes, and of the fears it produces. You need to know that with appropriate medications and care, especially today, the disease can be controlled. The severe destructive changes that can occur should become a rarity with our new medications. Beyond that you need the emotional support of a loving partner. You need to access the physical immune and hormonal benefits of a healthy sexual relationship.

Depression and anxiety reduce pain tolerance. Easing them can reduce the pain. The benefits of a warm sexual relationship and of alcohol used appropriately can ease anxiety and reduce depression and pain. When sex is difficult or painful, there are many things you can do to help. Focus on touch, sharing, and closeness. Find positions that are comfortable. Use pillows to support yourself or your partner. Use a lubricant. Bring your partner to orgasm without coitus. Most of all share the warmth of love. Touching and being touched are potent elements in a healthy sexual relationship. The skin is a major sex organ, and it responds with pleasure to stroking and caressing.

Start with a gentle massage. To break down barriers that have come between you, a light touch massage of the neck, the face, the back and the buttocks, legs and feet, arms and hands can be very pleasurable and non-threatening. This is a good beginning. Communicate with it and through it. Let your partner know what feels good. Let your partner know your love.

In order to understand how sex can affect arthritis, and to understand how our most valuable new drugs work, we need to understand something about inflammation and the mind, the nervous system, the immune system, and the endocrine system. All of these systems inter-relate and contribute to the symptoms and effects of arthritis and to the means of treating arthritis.

Over all of human history until the beginning of the 20th century, we had to rely on natural remedies alone. Some of them have beneficial therapeutic effects. Today our pharmaceutical researchers have identified the active ingredients of many of these natural remedies, have purified them, and improved them so now the more effective forms are used as our primary therapeutic agents. With our new knowledge, new designer drugs have been developed that are providing dramatic benefits. Now the natural or herbal preparations are considered complementary and alternative forms of therapy. Many alternative therapies have some merit. Some are not effective. Some can be dangerous. With all considered, after reviewing their effects on arthritis and on health in general, the ultimate in alternative therapies must be sex and alcohol.

BIBLIOGRAPHY

Alternative Therapies

Koenig H. Religion, Spirituality and Medicine: How are they related and what does it mean? Mayo Clinic Proc 2001; 76:1189-90

Mueller P, Plevak D, Rummans T. Religious involvement, spirituality, and medicine: implications for clinical practice. Mayo Clin Proc. 2001;76:1225-1235

Aviles J, Whelan E, Hernke D, Williams B, Kenny K, O'Fallon M, Kopecky S. Intercessory prayer and cardiovascular disease progression in a coronary care unit population:a randomized controlled trial. Mayo Clin Proc.2001;76:1192-98

Porter R. *Quacks Fakers & Charlatans in English Medicine*.2000; Tempus Publishing Inc. UK.

Adams F, Kelly E. The Genuine Works of Hippocrates. 1939 The Williams & Wilkins Company, publishers.

McCoy B. Quack Tales of medical fraud from the museum of questionable medical devices. 2000 Santa Monica Press.

Gilbert S. Medical fakes and frauds. 1989 Chelsea House Publishers. Pages 34, 15-24, 32-70.

Arthritis Foundation Pamphlet. Arthritis Unproven Remedies. 1987

Armstrong D, Armstrong E. The Great American Medicine Show. Prentice Hall 1991

Barrett S, Jarvis W. The Health Robbers. 1993 Promethius Books

Altman RD, Marcussen KC. Effects of a ginger extract on knee pain in patients with osteoarthritis. Arthritis Rheum.2001; 44:2531-8.

Reginster JY, Gillot V, Bruyere O, Henroitin Y. A randomized, placebo-controlled cross-over study of ginger extracts and ibuprofen in osteoarthritis. Curr Rheumatol Ret. 2000 2:472-7

Sharma JN. Suppressive effects of eugenol and ginger oil on arthritic rats. Pharmacology. 1994; 49:314-8.

Srivastava KC, Mustafa T. Ginger (Zingiber officinale) in rheumatism and musculoskeletal disorders.Med Hypotheses 1992;39:342-8

Reginster J, Deroisy R, Rovati L, Lee R, Lejeune E, Bruyere O, Giacovelli G, Henrotin Y, Dacre J, Gosset C. Long-term effects of glucosamine sulphate on osteoarthritis progression: a randomized, placebo-controlled clinical trial. The Lancet. 2001; 357:251-256

Pavelka K, Gatterova J, Olejarova M, Machacek S, Giacovelli G, Rovati L. Glucosamine sulfate use and delay of progression of knee osteoarthritis. Archives of Internal Medicine 2002; 162:2113-2123

McAlindon T. Glucosamine and chondroitin for osteoarthritis? Bull Rheum Dis. 2001;50:1-4

Drovanti A, Bignamini A, Rovati AL. Therapeutic activity of oral glucosamine sulfate in osteoarthritis. Clin Ther 1980; 7:104-9

Noack W, Fischer M, Forster KK, Rovati LC, Setnikar I. Glucosamine Sulfate in osteoarthritis of the knee. Osteoarthritis and Cartilage 1994; 2:51-9.

Mankin HJ, Johnson ME, Lippiello L. Biochemical and metabolic abnormalities in articular cartilage from osteoarthritis human hips. III Distribution and metabolism of amino sugar-containing macromolecules. J bone and Joint Surgery. 1981; 63-A: 131-9.

Malemud CJ, Shuckett R, Goldberg VM. Changes in proteogly-cans of human osteoarthritic cartilage maintained in explant culture; implications for understanding repair in osteoarthritis. Scand J Rheumatol Suppl;1988;77:7-12.

Bassleer C, Rovati I, Franchimont P. Stimulation of proteoglycan production by glucosamine sulfate in chondrocytes isolated from human osteoarthritic articular cartilage in vitro. Osteoarthritis Cartilage 1998;6:427-34.

Schwartz ER, Leveille CR, Stevens JW, Oh WH. Proteoglycan structure and metabolism in normal and osteoarthritic cartilage of guinea pigs Arthritis Rheum 1981;24:528-39

www.nutriteam.com/msm.htm

Pubmed.nl.com Medline search 5-25-2002.

Bradley JD, Flusser D, Katz BP, Schumacher HR Jr, Brandy KD, Chambers MA, Zonay LJ. A randomized double blind placebo controlled trial of intravenous loading with S-adenosylmethionine (SAM) followed by oral SAM therapy in patients with knee osteoarthritis.1994; 21:905-11.

Hirazumi A, Furusawa E. An immunomodulatory polysaccharide-rich substance from the fruit juice of Morinda citrifolia (noni) with antitumor activity. Phytother Res 1999; 13:380-7.

Arthritis Today. Sept-Oct 1991.

Panush RS, Carter RL, Katz P, Kowsari B, Longley S, Finnie S. Diet therapy for rheumatoid arthritis. Arthritis Rheum 1983;26:462-71

Pemberton RW. Insects and other arthropods used as drugs in Korean traditional medicine

Panush RS. Honeybees and arthritis: Sharpening perspective on a sticky issue. Rheumatology 1988; 15:1461-2.

Kraus A, Guerra-Bautista G, Alarcon-Segovia D. Salmonella Arizona arthritis and septicemia associated with rattlesnake ingestion by patients with connective tissue diseases. A dangerous complication of folk medicine. J Rheumatol 1991; 18:1328.

Waterman S, Juarez G, Carr SJ, Kilman L. Salmonella Arizona infections in Latinos associated with rattlesnake folk medicine. Am J Public Health 1990; 80:286-9.

Trentham DE. Oral tolerization as a treatment of rheumatoid arthritis. Rheum Dis Clin North Am 1998; 24:525-36.

Sieper J, Mitchison AN.Therapy with oral type II collagen as a new possibility of selective immunosuppression in therapy of rheumatoid arthritis. Z Rheumatol 1994; 53:53-8

Barnett ML, Kremer JM, St Clair EW, Clegg DO, Furst D, Weisman M, Fletcher MJ, Chasan-Taber S, Finger E, Morales A, Le CH, Trentham DE. Treatment of rheumatoid arthritis with oral type II collagen. Results of a multicenter, double-blind, placebo-controlled trial. Arthritis Rheum 1998; 42:585-7

Caldwell JR. Venoms, copper and zinc in the treatment of arthritis. Rheum Dis Clin N. Am. 1999;25:919-22.

Berman BM, Singh BB, Lao L, Langengerg P, Li H, Hadhazy V, Bareta J, Hochberg M. A randomized trial of acupuncture as an adjunctive therapy in osteoarthritis of the knee. Rheumatology 1999; 38:346-54.

Ernst E. Acupuncture as a symptomatic treatment of osteoarthritis. A systematic review. Scand J Rheumatol 1997; 26:444-7.

Acupuncture in patients with osteoarthritis pain; a placebo controlled study. Am J Chin Med 1991; 19:95-100.

Deluze C, Bosia L, Zirbs A, Chantraine A, Vischer TL. Electroacupuncture in fibromyalgia: results of a controlled trial. BMJ 1992; 305:1249-52.

Erickson, B The effects of low and very low doses of ionizing radiation on human health. Proceedings of the Consail Francais des Travailieurs du Nucleaire at the University of Versailles-Saint Quentin en Yvelines, June 17-18, 1999 Reprinted with permission of the author.

Hill S, Eckett M, Paterson, Harkness E. A pilot study to evaluate the effects of floatation spa treatment on patients with osteoarthritis. Complementary therapies in medicine.1999;p235-238

Arthritis and Sex

Twain M. Letters from the earth. Ed. By Bernard DeVoto. Perennial Library, Harper and Row, Publishers, New York.

Katz WA. Sexuality and Arthritis. Rheumatic Diseases:Diagnosis and management. J B Lippincott Co. Philadelphia 1977. 1011-1020.

Siegel BS. Love, medicine and miracles. Harper & Row, Publishers. New York 1986.

Kraaimaat FW, Bakker AH, Janssen E, Bijlsma JWJ. Intrusiveness of rheumatoid arthritis on sexuality in male and female patients living with a spouse. Arthritis Care and Research 1996; 9:120-5

Ferguson K, Figley B. Sexuality and rheumatic disease: a prospective study. Sex Disabil 1979; 2:130-8.

Yoshino S, Uchida S. Sexual problems of women with rheumatoid arthritis. Arch Phys Med Rehabil 1981; 62:122-3

Blake DL, Maisiak R, Alarcon GS, Holley HL, Brown S. Sexual quality-of-life of patients with arthritis compared to arthritis-free controls. J Rheumatol 1987; 14:570-6

Wise TN. Sexuality in chronic illness. Primary Care 1977; 4:199-208.

Kraaimaat FW, Rien MJ, Dam-Baggen V, Bijlsma JWJ. Association of social support and the spouse's reaction with psychological distress in male and female patients with rheumatoid arthritis. J Rheumatology 1995; 22:644-8.

Snelling J. The effect of chronic pain on the family unit. J Advanced Nursing. 1994; 19:543-51.

Editorial. Mental problems in Rheumatoid arthritis. BMJ 8 Nov 1969: 319

Currey HLF. Osteoarthrosis of the hip joint and sexual activity. Ann Rheum Dis. 1970; 29:488-93.

Manne SL, Zautra AJ. Spouse criticism and support: Their association with coping and psychological adjustment among women with rheumatoid arthritis. J Personality and social psychology 1989; 56:608-617.

Schwartz L, Slater MA, Birchler GR. The role of pain behaviors in the modulation of marital conflict in chronic pain couples. Pain.1996; 65: 227-233.

Schmoldt RA, Pope CR, Hibbard JH. Marital interaction and the health and well-being of spouses. Women and Health 1989; 15:35-56

Elst P, Sybesma T, Van Der Stadt RJ, Prins APA, Muller WH, Den Butter A. Sexual problems in rheumatoid arthritis and ankylosing spondylitis. Arthritis Rheum. 1984; 27:217-220.

Yocum DE, Castro WL, Cornett M. Exercise, education and behavioral modification as alternative therapy for pain and stress in rheumatic disease. Rheum Dis clin N Am 2000; 26:145-59.

Jorgensen C, Bressot N, Bologna C, Sany J. Dysregulation of the hypothalamo-pituitary axis in rheumatoid arthritis. J Rheumatol 1995; 22:1829-33.

SchedlowskiM, Wiechert D, Wagner T, Tewes U. Acute psychological stress increases plasma levels of cortisol, prolactin and TSH. Life Sciences 1992; 50:1201-5.

Schedlowski M, Fluge T, Richter S, Tewes U, Schmidt RE, Wagner T. B-Endorphin, but not substance-P, is increased by acute stress in humans. Psychoneuroendocrinology1995; 20:103-110.

Kruger THC, Haake P, Hartmnn U, Schedlowski M, Exton MS. Orgasm-induced prolactin secretion: feedback control of sexual drive? Neuroscience and Behavioral Rev 2002;26:31-44.

Zautra AJ, Hoffman J, Potter P, Matt KS, Yocum D, Castro L. Examination of changes in interpersonal stress as a factor in disease exacerbations among women with rheumatoid arthritis. Ann Behav Med 1997; 19:279-86.

Matt KS, Fairchild L, Nordensson, et al: neuroendocrine measures of stress reactivity in patients with rheumatoid arthritis (abstract). Clin Exp Rheumatol. 1998; 16:638.

Cornett M, Yocum DE, Castro WL, et al. Living healthy with arthritis: A community based pilot program focusing on wellness and preventive arthritis care through exercise, nutrition and a balanced lifestyle (abstract). Arthritis Rheum. 1998 Suppl; 41:S186.

Pike JL, Smith TL, Hauger RL, Nicassio PM, Patterson TL, McClintick J, Costlow C, Irwin MR. Chronic life stress alters sympathetic neuroendocrine and immune responsivity to an acute plychological stressor in humans. Psychosom Med 1997; 59:447-57.

Glaser R, Kiecolt-Glaser JK, Malarkey WB, Sheridan JF. The influence of plychological stress on the immune response to vaccines. Ann N Y Acad Sci 1998; 840;649-55

Pawlak CR, Jacobs R, Mikeska E, Ochsmann S, Lombardi MS, Kavelaars A,Heijnen CJ, Schmidy RE, Schedlowski M. Brain Behav Immun 1999; 13:287-302.

Exton MS, Bindert A, Kruger T, Scheller F, Hartmann U, Schedlowski M. Cardiovascular and endocrine alterations after masturbation-induced orgasm in women. Psychosom Med 1999; 61:280-9.

Turner RA, Altemus M, Enos T, Cooper B, McGuinness T. Preliminary research on plasma oxytocin in normal cycling women: investigating emotion and interpersonal distress. Psychiatry 1999; 62:97-113

Blaicher W, Gruber D, bieglmayer C, Blaicher AM, Knogler W, Huber JC. The role of oxytocin in relation to female sexual arousal. Gynecol Obstet Invest 1999; 47:125-6.

Uvnas-Moberg K. Oxytocin may mediate the benefits of positive social interaction and emotions. Psychoneuroendocrinoloty 1998; 23:819-35.

Murphy MF, Checkley SA, Seckl JR, Lightman SL. Naloxone inhibits oxytocin release at orgasm in man. J Clin Endocrinol Metab 1990; 71:1056-8

Carmichael MS, Warburton VL, DixenJ, Davidson JM. Relationships among cardiovascular, muscular, and oxytocin responses during human sexual activity. Arch Sex Behav 1994; 23:59-79 http://www.healthcentral.com/drdean/deanfulltesttopics.cfm?id-29239.

Jorgensen C, Bressot N, Bologna C, Sany J. Dysregulation of the hypothalamo-pituitary axis in rheumatoid arthritis. J Rheumatol 1995; 22:1829-33.

Hamilton A. Sexual problems in arthritis and allied conditions. International rehab Med. 1981; 3:38-42.

Shaul MP. From early twinges to mastery; the process of adjustment in living with rheumatoid arthritis. Arthritis Care and Research 1995; 8:290-7.

Westheimer R. Dr. Ruth's Guide to Good Sex. Warner Books, N Y. 1983.

Keillor Garrison, et al. A Prairie Home Companion Preet Good Jokes. High Bridge Company 1000 Westgate Drive. St. Paul, Minn. 5514

Paget Lou, How to be a great lover. Broadway Books, Random House. N Y 1999.

The Benefits of Alcohol

Goldberg DM, Soleas GJ, Levesque M. Moderate alcohol consumption: the gentle face of Janus. Clin Biochem 1999; 32:505-18.

Paolisso G, Valentini G, Giugliano D, Marrazzo G, Tirri R, Gallo M, Tirri G, Barricchio M, D'Onofiro F. Evidence for peripheral impaired glucose handling in patients with connective tissue diseases. Metabolism 1991; 40:902-7.

Svenson KL, Pollare T, Lithell H, Hallgren R. Impaired glucose handling in active rheumatoid arthritis: relationship to peripheral insulin resistance. Metabolism 1988; 37:125-30.

Dessein PH, Stanwix AE, Moomal Z. Rheumatoid arthritis and cardiovascular disease may share similar risk factors. Rheumatology (Oxford) 2001; 40:703-4.

Dessein PH, Joffe BI, Stanwix AE, Moomal Z. Hyposecretion of the adrenal androgen dehydroepiandrosterone sulfate and its relation to clinical variables in inflammatory arthritis. Arthritis Res. 2001; 3:183-8.

Bjornadal L, Baecklund E, Yin L, Granath F, Klareskog L, Ekbom A. Decreasing mortality in patients with rheumatoid arthritis: Results from a large population based cohort in Sweden, 1964-95. J Rheumatol 2002: 29:906-12.

Gabriel S, Crowson C, O'Fallon WM. Heart disease in rheumatoid arthritis. Arthritis Rheum 1998; 9(Suppl):S132.

Pincus T, Brooks R H, Callahan R F. Prediction of long-term mortality in patients with rheumatoid arthritis according to simple questionnaire and joint count measures. Ann Intern Med 1994; 120:26-34.

Manzi S, Wasko M. Inflammation-mediated rheumatic diseases and atherosclerosis. Ann Rheum Dis. 2000; 59:321-5.

Goodson, N. Coronary artery disease and rheumatoid arthritis. Curr Opin Rheum. 2002; 14:115-120.

Turesson C, O'Fallon WM, Crowson CS, Gabries SE, Matteson EL. Occurrence of estraarticular disease manifestations is associated with excess mortality in a community based cohort of patients with rheumatoid arthritis. J Rheumatol 2002; 29:62-7.

DeMaria AN. Relative resk of cardiovascular events in patients with rheumatoid arthritis. Am J Cardiol 2002; 89:33D-38D.

Desmeules M, Lagace C, Nagpal S, Badley E M. Arthritis and cardiovascular disease risk profiles among Canadians. Arthritis Rheum 2001; Suppl. 1065

Jonsson SW, Backman C, Johnson O, Karp K, Lundstrom E, Sundqvist KG, Dahlqvist SR. Increased prevalence of atherosclerosis in patients with medium term rheumatoid arthritis. J Rheumatol 2001; 28:2597-602

George J, Harats D, Gilburd B, Levy Y, Langevitz P, Shoenfeld Y. Atherosclerosis-related markers in systemic lupus erythematosus patients: the role of humoral immunity in enhanced atherogenesis. Lupus 1999; 8:220-226.

Puurunen M, Manttari M, Manninen V, Tenkanen L, Alfthan g, Ehnholm C, Vaarala O, Aho K, Palosuo T. Arch Intern Med.1994; 154:2605-9.

Charney P. Coronary artery disease in young women: the menstrual cycle and other risk factors. Ann Intern Med. 2001; 135:1002-4

Davies KJ. Oxidative stress: the paradox of aerobic life. Biochem Soc Symp 1995; 61:1-31.

Ward J. Free radicals, antioxidants and preventive geriatrics Aust Fam Physician 1994; 23:1297-301, 1305.

Bauerova K, Bezek A. Role of reactive oxygen and nitrogen species in etiopathogenesis of rheumatoid arthritis. Gen Physiol biophys 1999; 18:15-20.

Tak PP, Zvaifler NJ, Green DR, Firestein GS, Rheumatoid arthritis and p53: how oxidative stress might alter the course of inflammatory diseases. Immunol today 2000; 21:78-82

Aruoma OJ, Kaur H, Halliwell B. Oxygen free radicals and human diseases. J R Soc Health 1991; 111:172-7.

Suryaprabha P, Das UN, Ramesh G, Kumar KV, Kumar GS. Reactive oxygen species, lipid peroxides and essential fatty acids in patients with rheumatoid arthritis and systemic lupus erythematosus. Prostaglandins Leukot Essent Fatty Acids 19891; 43:251-5.

Sung J, Hong J, Kang H, Choi I, Lim S, Lee J, Seok J, Hur G. Methotrexate suppresses the interleukin-6 induced generation of reactive oxygen species in the synoviocytes of rheumatoid arthritis. Immunopharmacology 2000; 47:35-44.

Ruf JC. Wine and polyphenols related to platelet aggregation and atherothrombosis. Drugs Exp Clin Res 1999; 25:125-31.

LaPorte R, Valvo-Gerard L, Kuller L, Dai W, Bates M, Cresanta j, Williams K, Palkin D. The relationship between alcohol consumption, liver enzymes and high=density lipoprotein cholesterol. Circulation 1981; 64(Suppl III):68-72.

Agewall S, Wright S, Doughty RN, Whalley GA, Duxbury M, Sharpe N. Does a glass of red wine improve endothelial function? Eur Heart J 2000; 21:74-78.

Trevithick CC, Chartrand MM, Wahlman J, Rahman F, Hirst M, Trevithick JR. Shaken, not stirred: bioanalytical study of the antioxidant activities of martinis. BMJ 1999; 319:1600-2.

Stein JH, Keevil JG, Wiebe DA, Aeschlimann S, Folts JD. Purple grape juice improves endothelial function and reduces the susceptibility of LDL cholesterol to oxidation in patients with coronary artery disease. Circulation 1999; 100:1050-5.

Keevil JG,, Osman HE, Reed JD, Folts JD. Grape juice, but not orange juice or grapefruit juice, inhibits human platelet aggregation. J Nutr 2000; 130:53-6.

Croft KD. The chemistry and biological effects of flavonoids and phenolic acids. Ann N Y Acad Sci. 1998; 854:435-42.

Serafini M, Maiani G, Ferro-Luzzi A. Alcohol-free red wine enhances plasma antioxidant capacity in humans. J Nutr 1998; 128:1003-7.

Wiese JG, Shlipak MG, Browner WS. The alcohol hangover. Ann Intern Med 2000; 132:897-902.

Bondy SJ, Rehm J, Ashley MJ, Walsh G, Single E, Room R. Low=risk drinking guidelines: the scientific evidence. Rev Canadienne de Sante Publique 1999; 90:264-70.

Baum-Baicker c. The psychological benefits of moderate alcohol consumption: a review of the literature. Drug and Alcohol Dependence 1985; 15:305-22.

Gaiter DJ, Brecher J. Love By The Glass. Tasting notes from a marriage. Villard Books. Random House N Y. 2002

Johnson-Bell L. Pairing Wine and Food. A handbook for all cuisines. Burford Books. Short Hills, N J. 1999.

Joseph R. Good Wine Guide 2002.DK Publishers, a Penguin Company.